Céline Robert-Tissot

Resistance to Viral Infection by Stimulation of Innate Immunity

Céline Robert-Tissot

Resistance to Viral Infection by Stimulation of Innate Immunity

The Domestic Cat, Synthetic CpG Oligonucleotides and FIV Infection

Südwestdeutscher Verlag für Hochschulschriften

Impressum/Imprint (nur für Deutschland/ only for Germany)
Bibliografische Information der Deutschen Nationalbibliothek: Die Deutsche Nationalbibliothek
verzeichnet diese Publikation in der Deutschen Nationalbibliografie; detaillierte bibliografische
Daten sind im Internet über http://dnb.d-nb.de abrufbar.
Alle in diesem Buch genannten Marken und Produktnamen unterliegen warenzeichen-, marken-
oder patentrechtlichem Schutz bzw. sind Warenzeichen oder eingetragene Warenzeichen der
jeweiligen Inhaber. Die Wiedergabe von Marken, Produktnamen, Gebrauchsnamen,
Handelsnamen, Warenbezeichnungen u.s.w. in diesem Werk berechtigt auch ohne besondere
Kennzeichnung nicht zu der Annahme, dass solche Namen im Sinne der Warenzeichen- und
Markenschutzgesetzgebung als frei zu betrachten wären und daher von jedermann benutzt
werden dürften.

Verlag: Südwestdeutscher Verlag für Hochschulschriften Aktiengesellschaft & Co. KG
Dudweiler Landstr. 99, 66123 Saarbrücken, Deutschland
Telefon +49 681 37 20 271-1, Telefax +49 681 37 20 271-0, Email: info@svh-verlag.de
Zugl.: Zurich, Vetsuisse Faculty, University of Zurich, Diss., 2008

Herstellung in Deutschland:
Schaltungsdienst Lange o.H.G., Berlin
Books on Demand GmbH, Norderstedt
Reha GmbH, Saarbrücken
Amazon Distribution GmbH, Leipzig
ISBN: 978-3-8381-0655-7

Imprint (only for USA, GB)
Bibliographic information published by the Deutsche Nationalbibliothek: The Deutsche
Nationalbibliothek lists this publication in the Deutsche Nationalbibliografie; detailed
bibliographic data are available in the Internet at http://dnb.d-nb.de.
Any brand names and product names mentioned in this book are subject to trademark, brand or
patent protection and are trademarks or registered trademarks of their respective holders. The
use of brand names, product names, common names, trade names, product descriptions etc.
even without a particular marking in this works is in no way to be construed to mean that such
names may be regarded as unrestricted in respect of trademark and brand protection legislation
and could thus be used by anyone.

Publisher:
Südwestdeutscher Verlag für Hochschulschriften Aktiengesellschaft & Co. KG
Dudweiler Landstr. 99, 66123 Saarbrücken, Germany
Phone +49 681 37 20 271-1, Fax +49 681 37 20 271-0, Email: info@svh-verlag.de

Copyright © 2009 by the author and Südwestdeutscher Verlag für Hochschulschriften
Aktiengesellschaft & Co. KG and licensors
All rights reserved. Saarbrücken 2009

Printed in the U.S.A.
Printed in the U.K. by (see last page)
ISBN: 978-3-8381-0655-7

Table of contents

1 Summary 1

2 Introduction 3

3 Literature 7
  3.1 FIV Literature Overview 7
    3.1.1 Viral Morphology and Genetic Structure 7
    3.1.2 Viral Life Cycle 10
      3.1.2.1 Receptor Usage and Cell Entry 10
      3.1.2.2 Cellular Tropism 11
      3.1.2.3 Replication and Production of Infectious Virions 12
    3.1.3 Pathogenesis 14
      3.1.3.1 Viral Transmission 14
      3.1.3.2 Course of Disease 15
      3.1.3.3 Immunological Aspects 17
        3.1.3.3.1 CD4+ T Lymphocyte Depletion 17
        3.1.3.3.2 CD8+ T Lymphocyte Anti-Viral Activity 18
        3.1.3.3.3 T Cell Dysfunction, Anergy and Apoptosis 19
        3.1.3.3.4 Cytokine Production 20
        3.1.3.3.5 Antibody Responses 22
    3.1.4 Epidemiology 23
      3.1.4.1 Viral Clades 23
      3.1.4.2 Host Range 24
      3.1.4.3 Occurrence and Prevalence Studies 25
    3.1.5 Clinical Aspects 26
    3.1.6 Diagnostic Approach 30

Table of contents

3.1.7 Treatment	33
3.1.8 Prevention	39
3.1.8.1 General Considerations	39
3.1.8.2 Vaccination	40
3.1.8.2.1 Choice of Adjuvant	41
3.1.8.2.2 Importance of Challenge Methods	44
3.1.8.2.3 Immune Correlates of Protection and Passive Immunity	46
3.1.8.2.4 FIV Vaccine Trials	47
3.1.8.2.4.1 Generalities	47
3.1.8.2.4.2 Conventional Vaccines	49
3.1.8.2.4.3 Subunit Vaccines	54
3.1.8.2.4.4 DNA Vaccines	59
3.1.8.2.5 Enhancement Problem	62
3.2 CpG Oligonucleotide Literature Overview	66
3.2.1 Insight on Innate Immunity and Toll-like Receptors	67
3.2.2 Definition of CpGs and Natural Occurrence	70
3.2.3 Uptake Mechanisms and Signal Transduction	71
3.2.4 Immunological Effects of CpGs	75
3.2.4.1 Cellular Immunomodulation of CpG DNA	76
3.2.4.1.1 B Cells	77
3.2.4.1.2 Dendritic Cells	78
3.2.4.1.3 Monocytes and Macrophages	79
3.2.4.1.4 Natural Killer Cells	80
3.2.4.1.5 T Cells	81
3.2.4.1.6 Neutrophils	82
3.2.4.2 Creation of a Th1-like Cytokine Milieu	82
3.2.4.3 Production of IFN-α	83
3.2.5 Species Specificity in CpG DNA Recognition	85
3.2.6 Production of Synthetic Oligonucleotides	87
3.2.7 Immunotherapeutic Possibilities	89
3.2.7.1 Protection of Immunocomprimised Hosts	89

3.2.7.2 Cancer	91
3.2.7.3 Allergy	94
3.2.7.4 Infectious Diseases	96
3.2.7.4.1 Bacterial and Parasitical Infections	97
3.2.7.4.2 Viral Infections	98
3.2.7.5 Use of CpG ODN as Vaccine Adjuvants	102
3.2.7.6 Safety Concerns	105

4 Material and Methods — 109

4.1 Objectives	109
4.2 General Information and Important Methods	110
4.2.1 Enzyme-linked Immunosorbent Assay	110
4.2.2 Nucleic Acid Extractions	111
4.2.3 Real-Time Fluorogenic Polymerase Chain Reaction	112
4.2.4 Peripheral Blood Mononuclear Cell Isolation	114
4.3 Pre-experiment Formalities	116
4.3.1 Cats	116
4.3.2 Adaptation Period and Assessment of Health Status	117
4.4 Course of the Study	118
4.4.1 Treatment Protocol	119
4.4.2 Challenge Infection	120
4.4.3 Clinical Auscultations, Blood and Oropharyngeal Swab Collections	121
4.4.4 Laboratory Analyses of Relevant Host and Viral Parameters	121
4.4.4.1 Haematology and Clinical Chemistry	121
4.4.4.2 Evaluation of Host Immune Parameters	122
4.4.4.2.1 Seroconversion	122
4.4.4.2.2 Determination of Cytokine Expression	122
4.4.4.2.2.1 Cytokine Measurements in Whole Blood	123
4.4.4.2.2.2 Cytokine Measurements in Stimulated and Unstimulated PBMCs	124
4.4.4.3 Evolution of FIV Infection	125
4.4.4.3.1 Measurements of Proviral and Viral Loads in Blood	125

Table of contents

  4.4.4.3.2 Isolation of Virus from Plasma — 126
  4.4.4.3.3 Measurements of Viral Load in Saliva — 127
 4.5 Statistical Analysis — 127

5 Results — 129

 5.1 Clinical Examination — 130
  5.1.1 Body Weight — 130
  5.1.2 Body Temperature — 130
  5.1.3 Clinical Symptoms — 131
 5.2 Haematology — 132
  5.2.1 Red Blood Cell Parameters — 133
  5.2.2 White Blood Cell Parameters — 134
   5.2.2.1 Absolute White Blood Cell Counts — 134
   5.2.2.2 Neutrophilic and Eosinophilic Granulocytes — 135
   5.2.2.3 Monocytes — 136
   5.2.2.4 Lymphocytes — 137
 5.3 Clinical Chemistry — 138
  5.3.1 Substrates — 138
  5.3.2 Enzymes — 139
  5.3.3 Electrolytes — 140
 5.4 Immunology — 142
  5.4.1 Antibodies to FIV TM — 142
  5.4.2 Cytokine Measurements — 143
   5.4.2.1 Cytokine Expression in Whole Blood — 143
   5.4.2.2 Stimulation of Cytokine Production *in vitro* — 145
 5.5 Evaluation of Viral Infection — 148
  5.5.1 FIV Proviral Loads in Whole Blood — 148
  5.5.2 FIV Viral Loads — 149
   5.5.2.1 FIV Viral Loads in Plasma — 149
   5.5.2.2 FIV Viral Loads in Saliva — 150
  5.5.3 Isolation of Virus from Plasma — 152

6 Discussion — 155
6.1 Background of the Study — 155
6.2 Design of the Study — 158
6.3 Relevant Results — 162
6.3.1 Results of the Clinical Examinations — 162
6.3.2 Blood Parameters — 164
6.3.2.1 Haematology — 164
6.3.2.1.1 Deviation in Red Blood Cell Parameters — 164
6.3.2.1.1.1 Hematocrit — 164
6.3.2.1.2 Deviation in White Blood Cell Parameters — 165
6.3.2.1.2.1 Leucocytes — 165
6.3.2.1.2.2 Neutrophilic Granulocytes — 165
6.3.2.1.2.3 Eosinophilic Granulocytes — 166
6.3.2.1.2.4 Monocytes — 166
6.3.2.1.2.5 Lymphocytes — 167
6.3.2.2 Clinical Chemistry — 167
6.3.2.2.1 Substrates — 167
6.3.2.2.1.1 Blood Glucose Levels — 167
6.3.2.2.1.2 Blood Urea Levels — 169
6.3.2.2.2 Enzymes — 169
6.3.2.2.2.1 Lipase — 169
6.3.2.2.2.2 ALAT — 169
6.3.2.2.3 Electrolytes — 170
6.3.2.2.3.1 Blood Chloride Levels — 170
6.3.2.2.3.2 Blood Phosphorus Levels — 170
6.3.3 Evaluation of Viral Infection — 170
6.3.3.1 FIV Proviral Loads in Whole Blood — 171
6.3.3.2 FIV Viral Loads — 172
6.3.3.2.1 FIV Viral Loads in Plasma — 172
6.3.3.2.2 FIV Viral Loads in Saliva — 173
6.3.3.3 Isolation of Virus from Plasma — 174

Table of contents

    6.3.4 Immunological Measurements — 176
        6.3.4.1 Anti-TM ELISA — 178
        6.3.4.2 Cytokine Measurements — 178
            6.3.4.2.1 Cytokine Expression in Whole Blood — 179
            6.3.4.2.2 Stimulation of Cytokine Expression *in vitro* — 180
  6.4 Conclusion and Future Perspectives — 183

7 References — *187*

8 Acknowledgements — *215*

Index

Figures

Figure 1 : Structure of FIV	8
Figure 2 : FIV genome	10
Figure 3 : FIV replication cycle	14
Figure 4 : Course of viremia, antibody production, CD4+ and CTL in FIV infection	17
Figure 5 : Phylogenetic tree of FIV subtypes	24
Figure 6 : Mechanisms of antibody-dependent enhancement	64
Figure 7 : Signalling cascade following trigger of TLR9	74
Figure 8 : Immunostimulatory effects of TLR9 activation in B cells and pDCs	84
Figure 9 : Principles of real-time PCR	114
Figure 10 : PBMC isolation by Ficoll-Hypaque® gradient	116
Figure 11 : Schedule of the study	119
Figure 12 : Schematic representation of the dSLIM™ molecule	119
Figure 13 : Mean body weights	131
Figure 14 : Mean body temperatures	131
Figure 15 : Mean red blood cell counts	133
Figure 16 : Mean hematocrit values	134
Figure 17 : Mean white blood cell counts	134
Figure 18 : Mean absolute neutrophilic granulocyte counts	136
Figure 19 : Mean absolute eosinophilic granulocyte counts	136
Figure 20 : Mean absolute lymphocyte counts	137
Figure 21 : Mean absolute monocyte counts	137
Figure 22 : Mean blood glucose levels	138
Figure 23 : Mean blood urea levels	139
Figure 24 : Mean blood lipase levels	140
Figure 25 : Mean blood alanin-aminotransferase levels	141

Index

Figure 26 : Mean blood chloride levels — 141
Figure 27 : Mean blood phosphorus levels — 142
Figure 28 : Mean serum anti-TM antibody levels — 144
Figure 29 : Mean GAPDH mRNA expression in whole blood — 144
Figure 30 : Mean IL-10 mRNA expression in whole blood — 145
Figure 31 : Mean IL-12 p40 mRNA expression in whole blood — 147
Figure 32 : Mean GAPDH mRNA expression of isolated PBMCs — 147
Figure 33 : Mean IL-10 mRNA expression of isolated PBMCs — 148
Figure 34 : Mean IL-12 p40 mRNA expression of isolated PBMCs — 148
Figure 35 : Mean FIV proviral loads — 149
Figure 36 : Mean FIV viral loads in plasma — 150
Figure 37 : Mean FIV viral loads in saliva — 151
Figure 38 : Individual FIV viral loads in saliva — 151
Figure 39 : Individual infectious FIV isolation — 152

Tables

Table 1 : Structural proteins and enzymes of FIV — 9
Table 2 : FIV prevalence studies — 26
Table 3 : Clinical symptoms of stages of FIV infection — 27
Table 4 : Opportunistic pathogens observed in FIV infection — 29
Table 5 : Whole-virus and infected-cell vaccine trials against FIV infection — 52
Table 6 : Subunit vaccine trials against FIV infection — 56
Table 7 : DNA vaccine trials against FIV infection — 60
Table 8 : Breadth of the CpG-induced immune response — 85
Table 9 : Classes of CpG ODN — 89
Table 10 : Recent clinical studies using CpG ODN — 93
Table 11 : Application of CpG ODN in the context of infectious diseases — 100
Table 12 : Administration protocol of dSLIM™ *in vivo* — 120

Abreviations

A	Adenosine
ADCC	Antibody-dependent cellular cytotoxicity
ADE	Antibody-dependent enhancement
AIC	Amb a1/ immunostimulatory DNA conjugate
AIDS	Aquired immunodeficiency syndrome
ALAT	Alanin-aminotransferase
ALVAC	Recombinant canarypoxvirus
Amb a1	Ragweed pollen immunodominant allergen
AP	Alcaline phosphatase
APC	Antigen-presenting cell
ARC	AIDS-related complex
ASAT	Aspartate-aminotransferase
AZT	Azidothymidine
BCR	B cell antigen receptor
C	Cytosine
CA	Capsid protein
CCR	Chemokine (C-C motif) receptor
CD	Clusters of Differentiation
cDNA	Complementary DNA
CFA	Complete Freund's adjuvant
CID	Cat infectious dose
CNS	Central nervous system
Con A	Concanavalin A
CpG	Cytosine-phosphate-Guanine
CRFK	Crandell-Rees feline kidney
CSP	Malaria protein
CTL	Cytotoxic T lymphocyte

Abreviations

CTLA	Cytotoxic T lymphocyte antigen
DC	Dendritic cell
DNA	Deoxyribonucleic acid
EDTA	Ethylenediaminetetraacetic acid
EIAV	Equine infectious anemia virus
ELISA	Enzyme-linked immunosorbant assay
env	Envelope protein
FCoV	Feline coronavirus
FCS	Feotal calf serum
FCV	Feline calicivirus
Fe	Feline
FeLV	Feline leukemia virus
FHV	Feline herpes virus
FIV	Feline immunodeficiency virus
FPV	Feline parvovirus
FV	Friend virus
G	Guanosine
gag	Group-specific antigen
GAPDH	Glyceraldehyde 3-phosphate dehydrogenase
GMCSF	Granulocyte macrophage colony stimulating factor
gp	Glycoprotein
HAART	Highly active antiretroviral therapy
HBSS	Hanks' Balanced Salt Solution
HIV	Human immunodeficiency virus
HRP	Horse-radish peroxidase
HSV	Herpes simplex virus
Hu	Human
IFA	Incomplete freund's adjuvant
IFAI	Indirect fluorescent antibody immunoassay
IFN	Interferon
IL	Interleukin
IN	Integrase
IRAK	IL receptor-associated kinase

Abreviations

ISCOM	Immune-stimulating complex
LPS	Lipopolysaccharide
LTR	Long terminal repeat
MA	Matrix protein
MAP	Mitogen-activated protein
MCHC	Mean cell hemoglobin concentration
MDP	Muramyl dipeptide peptidoglycan
MGP	Magnetic bead particles
MHC	Major histocompatibility complex
MIDGE	Minimalistic immunogenic-defined gene expression
mRNA	Messenger RNA
MyD	Myeloid diferenciation primary response protein
NC	Nucleocapsid protein
NF-κB	Nuclear factor kappa B
NK	Natural killer
NNRTI	Non-nucleoside reverse transcriptase inhibitor
NRTI	Nucleoside reverse transcriptase inhibitor
OD	Optical density
ODN	Oligodeoxynucleotide
orf-A	Open reading frame A
OVA	Ovalbumin
PAMP	Pathogen-associated molecular pattern
PBMC	Peripheral blood mononuclear cell
PBS	Phosphate-buffered saline
pDC	Plasmacytoid dendritic cell
PI	Protease inhibitors
PID	Principal immunodominant domain
pODN	ODN with phosphodiester linkage
pol	Polymerase
PR	Protease
PRR	Pathogen recognition receptor
r	Recombinant
RBC	Red blood cell

Abreviations

rev	Regulator of virion protein expression	
RNA	Ribonucleic acid	
ROS	Reactive oxygen species	
RPMI	Roswell Park Memorial Institute medium	
RRE	*rev*-responsive element	
RT	Reverse transcriptase	
SAF	Syntex adjuvant formulation	
SARS	Severe acute immunodeficiency syndrome	
SDF	Stromal cell-derived factor	
SE	Salmonella enteritidis	
SMP	Streptavidin-coated magnetic beads	
sODN	ODN with phophorothioate linkage	
spf	Specific pathogen free	
SU	Surface glycoprotein	
T	Thymine	
TAB	TAK-binding protein	
TAK	TGF-activated kinase	
tat	Transactivator	
TGF	Transforming growth factor	
Th	T lymphocyte helper	
TIR	TLR/IL-R combination	
TLR	Toll-like receptor	
TM	Transmembrane protein	
TNA	Total nucleic acids	
TNF	Tumor necrosis factor	
TRAF	TNF receptor-associated factor	
Treg	T regulatory lymphocytes	
Trp	Tryptophan	
VEE	Venezuelan equine encephalitis	
vif	Viral infectivity factor	
VN	Virus neutralizing	
vpr	Virus protein R	
WBC	White blood cell	

1. Summary

This project was designed to study the *in vivo* immunomodulatory effects of CpG-containing oligonucleotides in the domestic cat and to determine their potential to induce short-term protection against FIV infection.
The prophylactic treatment of the cats was carried out with dSLIM™, a non-coding DNA molecule containing several unmethylated CpG motifs, previously shown to induce strong cellular immune responses and production of IFN-α, both highly desirable in the combat against viral infections.
A group of 10 spf cats was treated during 5 consecutive days; a second group, equally of 10 spf cats, was simultaneously treated with a placebo. Both groups were challenge infected with FIV 24 hours after the end of the treatment. Clinical and immunological parameters were closely monitored in the cats throughout the experiment.
When compared to the cats of the control group, 2 individuals treated with dSLIM™ indicated a 3-week delay in detection of proviral and viral loads in blood as well as isolation of infectious virus from plasma. A cytokine pattern representative of deviation to Th1 immune responses after treatment, as well as comparatively low antibody production after challenge enabled to attribute the partial resistance observed in these cats to cellular mechanisms.
Despite promising results in this study, further investigations are necessary to determine the feasibility of stimulation of innate immunity as alternative to the development of a vaccine against FIV.

2. Introduction

First isolated from a domestic cat (*Felis catus*) by Pedersen and colleagues in 1986, the *Feline Immunodeficiency* virus (FIV) is a retrovirus of the genus lentivirus, which causes progressive loss of CD4+ T lymphocytes in infected individuals. FIV disease persists lifelong, and most infected cats eventually succumb due to direct viral effects or, more commonly, to secondary infections resulting from virus-induced immunosuppression. Although the occurrence of infection in Switzerland remains relatively low, FIV is considered a main source of viral disease in stray and pet cat populations worldwide, with an overall prevalence of approximately 11%.

Among retroviral diseases affecting non-primate vertebrates, FIV infection in the cat is considered to be the closest model of *Human Immunodeficiency* virus (HIV) infection and acquired immunodeficiency syndrome (AIDS). Indeed, human HIV/AIDS and disease induced by FIV in cats not only share many biological and clinical properties, but host-virus immunological interactions indicate high similarities. Moreover, the diversity of primary FIV strains can be exploited to mirror the range of disease manifestations associated with HIV infection. The FIV model thus offers the opportunity to study lentiviral infection and immunopathology in natural, out-bred hosts, and enables valuable evaluation of preventive and therapeutic approaches to AIDS in both human and veterinary medicine.

Elaborating specific medical care or prevention methods against HIV and FIV infections has proven to be particularly tricky, as these viruses are very susceptible to evolutionary genetic alterations and possess highly developed adaptation faculties. Thus, simple mutational alterations result in resistant strains, considerably limiting the potential of existing antiviral drugs, and rendering prophylactic measures especially important in the combat against such viruses. However, the development

Introduction

of an effective vaccine is limited by the genetic and phenotypic diversities of these viruses in the field, and the numerous attempts to the development of specific prophylactic protection have unfortunately to date not indicated satisfying results. Stimulation of innate immunity represents an alternative method to specific immunization. Indeed, in the last 10 to 15 years, scientists have shown growing interest in better understanding the complexity of the innate immune system. It became rapidly clear that stimulation of the organism's first line of defence could be exploited to enhance short term resistance to a variety of infections. Innate immunity not only initiates immediate reaction to a wide range of pathogens, but greatly supports the subsequent development of a specific immune response.

Cytosine-phosphate-guanosine (CpG) dinucleotides are unmethylated and frequently present in bacterial DNA, whereas they are under-represented and selectively methylated in vertebrate genomes. Due to these differences, a non-self pattern recognition mechanism has evolved in vertebrate innate immune systems enabling them to counter invading pathogens. The early recognition of CpG DNA molecules by the immune system relies on Toll-like receptor 9 (TLR9), an ancient pattern recognition receptor (PRR) present in the main effector cells of innate immunity. Triggering of this receptor initiates intracellular cascades of events, enabling the expression of specific genes, thus leading to the induction of broad antimicrobial mechanisms. The most important response to activation of TLR9-linked mechanisms is probably the production of interferon-α (IFN-α), a type I IFN which happens to be a potent antiviral agent. IFN-α not only activates a wide variety of effector immune cell populations involved in both the first reaction to invading organisms and the mounting of a subsequent adaptive immune response, but induces, in yet uninfected cells, the synthesis of various proteins including enzymes, signaling proteins, antigen-presenting proteins and transcription factors, which specifically interfere with proper viral replication. Thus, by initiating potent mechanisms against viral dissemination, IFN-α altogether plays a major role in the induction of a global «antiviral state».

In recent years, great interest has been attributed to the development of diverse synthetic analogues of CpG-containing bacterial DNA, capable of inducing similar immune responses. Relative ease in the production and modulation of such synthetic compounds as well as early promising results of *in vitro* and *in vivo* experimentations rapidly rendered synthetic immunomodulatory CpG oligonucleotides (ODNs) particularly interesting in terms of prophylactic and therapeutic use for many diseases. In fact, synthetic CpG-containing molecules have gained such popularity in medical research, that current human clinical trials involve various types of cancer, allergies, as well as a broad range of infectious disease settings.

Due to the domestic cat's ancestral solitary way of life, feline viruses have developed very efficient transmission strategies to infect new hosts upon the rare contact between individuals, as well as the capability to induce latent and/or asymptomatic infections of the carrier cat. Although modern civilisation has considerably changed the living habits of the domestic cat populations, feline viruses, including FIV, have conserved their opportunistic behaviour throughout evolution. As a consequence, infections with viruses adapted to the domestic cat readily affect every individual living in a group. This most likely explains the very high frequency and importance of FIV, among other feline viral infections, observed in catteries and shelters, where cats from different backgrounds have narrow contact with each other. Agents capable of transiently conferring resistance to viral infection would be highly desirable to temporarily protect cats in such situations with increased risks of infection.

Targeting the innate immune system with highly selective synthetic CpG molecules seemingly offers a powerful means to enhance a broad spectrum antiviral resistance in the host. It was the aim of the present work to study *in vivo*, using the FIV model, the potential of a synthetic compound containing CpG motifs to confer short term resistance against viral infection. Elaboration of preventive measures against this feline virus appears particularly challenging, and promising results would create an exciting new opening for the development of novel short term antiviral preventive measures in both human and veterinary medicine.

3. Literature

3.1 FIV Literature Overview

Various publications concerning the *Feline Immunodeficiency* virus (FIV) have been highlighted in the dissertations of Kim Bauer (1994), Christian Leutenegger (1995) and Felicitas Boretti (1999). Besides important general aspects of FIV discussed in the early years after discovery of the virus, this work will mainly focus on the more recent studies aiding further characterization and understanding of FIV infection.

3.1.1 Viral Morphology and Genomic Structure

First discovered in California by Pedersen and colleagues in 1986, FIV is a typical lentivirus of the family retroviridae. Mature viral particles are spherical to ellipsoid, measure slightly over 100 nm in diameter, and present few, short spikes on the outer side of their envelope [1]. FIV virions contain two copies of a positive sense ribonucleic acid (RNA). Of approximately 10 kB in length, the FIV genome presents several typical characteristics of the retrovirus family. First, it contains from 5' to 3' three standard genes, *gag, pol, env,* that encode for proteins essential to viral structure and replication [2]:

1) *gag* (group specific antigen): encodes for the viral matrix (MA), capsid (CA) and nucleocapsid (NC) proteins
2) *pol* (polymerase): encodes for specific enzymes, including reverse transcriptase (RT), protease (PR), integrase (IN), and dUTPase
3) *env* (envelope): encodes for retroviral coat proteins designated as surface glycoprotein (SU) and transmembrane polyprotein (TM)

Literature

Additionally, the genome is flanked at each end by repeated sequences called long terminal repeats (LTR), comprised of untranslated 3' (U3, promoter/enhancer elements), repeat (R) and untranslated 5' (U5) regions. General functions of LTR include insertion of the viral genetic information in the host's cellular genome and enhancement of its transcription. Moreover, mutational analyzes have revealed numerous elements in the LTR U3 region such as AP-1, AP-4, ATF and NF1 binding sites, which constitute promoter sequences influencing viral gene expression [3]. Recent studies have also described elements both within U5 and the 5' end of gag, which are required for efficient packaging of newly produced FIV, thus allowing expansion of infection in the host [4]. Figures 1 and 2 are schematic representations of the FIV viral particle and the FIV genomic structure.

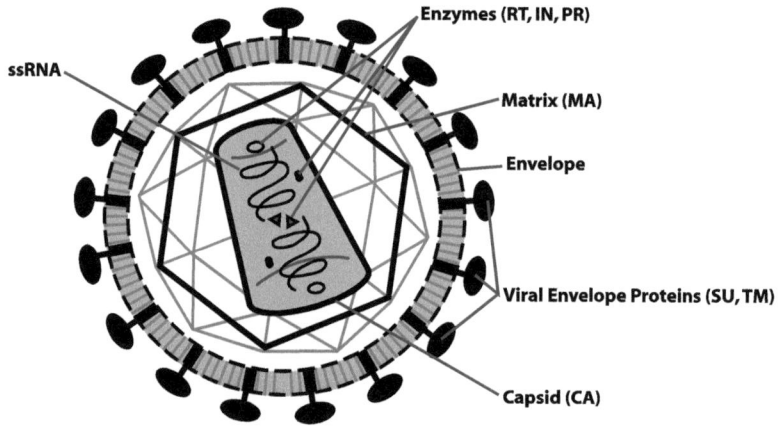

Figure 1: Structure of the feline immunodeficiency virus

Abreviation	Protein	Function	Genetic Origin
MA	Matrix	lines viral envelope	gag
CA	Capsid	protects viral core	
PR	Protease	*gag* protein cleavage during maturation	pol
RT	Reverse Transcriptase	reverse transcribes RNA genome	
IN	Integrase	Integration of provirus	
SU	Surface Glycoprotein	decorates outer envelope / major viral Ag	lines viral envelope
TM	Transmembrane Protein	inner component of mature viral envelope	

Table 1: Main structural proteins and enzymes of FIV, their functions and genetic origins

Other important regulatory genes of the FIV genome, shared with all or only certain members of the retrovirus family, include a *rev* gene (regulator of virion protein expression), a *vif* gene (viral infectivity factor), and an *orf-2* gene (also designated *orf-A*). *Rev* is vital for replication and packaging of all lentiviruses. Its translated protein acts as transporter of viral messenger RNA (mRNA) from nuclear localization to the cytoplasm, after interaction with a viral factor, the *rev*-responsive element (RRE) [5]. Most known lentiviruses include a *vif* gene, coding a viral infectivity factor responsible for production of infectious viral particles in producer cells and spread of infection to new target cells or tissues [6]. FIV transactivation was earlier thought to be dependent on *orf-2*, a short fragment placed within the vif sequence, with characteristics similar to those of the *tat* (transactivator) gene of the ungulate lentiviruses [7]. Interestingly, unlike other lentiviral transactivators, FIV *orf-2* was reported to require additional LTR elements for transactivation [8]. Moreover, recent studies indicated that *orf-2* function is involved in multiple steps of the FIV life cycle including both virion formation and infectivity [9]. The possibility that *orf-2* function resembles the *vpr* accessory genes of other lentiviruses rather than *tat*, is currently discussed.

Literature

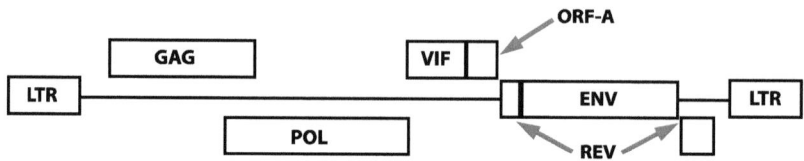

Figure 2: Schematic representation of the FIV genome

3.1.2 Viral Life Cycle

3.1.2.1 Receptor Usage and Cell Entry

FIV replication is similar to that of other retroviruses. The first essential step for effective infection of the target cell is the attachment of the virion to the cell surface. For efficient binding, viral surface glycoproteins and receptors of the outer cellular membrane both play an important role. Unlike the *Human Immunodeficiency* virus (HIV), the CD4 molecule is not used by the feline virus as primary receptor or co-receptor [10]. CD9 was earlier thought to be a main receptor for FIV, but further studies have demonstrated that antibodies directed against CD9 block virus release rather than viral entry [11].

With reference to knowledge on receptor usage by HIV, importance of chemokine receptors as means of target cell entry by FIV were more deeply studied. FIV was soon shown to utilize CXCR4 as a receptor for *env*-mediated fusion, and both primary as well as laboratory-adapted strains proved to need the receptor for host cell infection [12]. Further studies identified the second extracellular loop of CXCR4 as the primary determinant of target cell infection by FIV [13]. Moreover, *in vitro* FIV infection was shown to be inhibited by two different CXCR4 ligands, stromal cell derived factor 1 alpha (SDF1α) [14] and the bicyclam, AMD3100 [15]. However, some CXCR4 positive cell lines were resistant to FIV infection indicating the probable role of an additional receptor. The use of other chemokine receptors, such as CCR5 and CCR3 has also been demonstrated, as antibodies against CCR3 as well as RANTES, a ligand to CCR5, were able to inhibit FIV infection of target cells [16].

Literature

The recent identification of CD134, a T cell antigen and co-stimulatory molecule as primary receptor for FIV represents a tremendous step in the understanding of FIV interactions with its target cells [17]. CD134 expression was demonstrated to promote viral binding and render cells permissive for viral entry, but productive infection remained CXCR4 dependent. The tropism of FIV *in vivo* seems to be consistent with the predicted expression of CD134.

Viral characteristics critical for fusion with target cells appear to rely on a limited number of regions of the surface and transmembrane glycoproteins. The V3 loop of the viral SU glycoprotein 120 (gp120) has been shown to be critical for viral binding [18], and the V3-V5 region mediates chemokine receptor use [19]. Additionally, a tryptophan-rich motif, present membrane-proximally in the ectodomain of the FIV TM glycoprotein, proved to be essential in the processes of fusion and viral entry [20].

3.1.2.2 Cellular Tropism

The set of receptors present on the target cell surface determine the ability of FIV to gain entry into the cell and establish productive infection.

In vivo, FIV replicates in CD4+ and CD8+ T lymphocytes [21], B lymphocytes [22], macrophages [23], monocytes [24] and in astrocytes and microglia [25]. Some strains replicate preferentially in lymphoctytes (lymphocytotropic strains) and only minimally in monocytes, while other strains are able to replicate equally well in both cell types (monocytotropic strains). Moreover, certain strains have been shown to replicate in Kupffer cells [26], suggesting that these cells may play a role in the pathophysiology of FIV infection.

In vitro, the cellular tropism of primary isolates is restricted to mitogen-activated peripheral blood mononuclear cells (PBMCs), dendritic cells (DCs), macrophages and thymocytes. Tissue culture adapted strains can infect a wide range of cell types. In this way, various IL-2 dependent or independent T lymphblastoid cell lines have proven to satisfyingly simulate *in vivo* cytokine and major histocompatibility complex (MHC) class II molecule expression [27]. Only one T lymphoblastoid cell line, obtained from a specific pathogen free (spf) cat and characterized as Pan T+, CD4-, CD8-, was described to show a cytopathic effect upon inoculation with FIV [28]. Adapted strains can replicate in fibroblastoid cell lines, the most commonly used being Crandell-Rees Feline Kidney (CRFK) cells.

Interestingly, a human lymphoblastoid cell line [29], as well as human PBMCs [30], have efficiently been infected with FIV, but failure in the transcription step of replication caused latency of the virus in these cells. Infection of human cells by FIV was the first evidence of shared chemokine receptor use between primate and non-primate lentiviruses [31]. This finding represented a relevant step in the further knowledge of AIDS pathogenesis. Indeed, as FIV induces an immunodeficiency in the cat similar to AIDS in humans without using CD4 as a primary receptor for infection, the interaction between the virus and the chemokine receptor becomes a critical determinant of the pathogenesis of AIDS.

3.1.2.3 Replication and Production of Infectious Virions

After fusion of external viral and cellular proteins and FIV penetration of the cell, the viral core is freed in the cytoplasm and simultaneously undergoes specific structural changes (uncoating). The retroviral RNA within the modified core is reverse transcribed by the viral RT to a linear double-stranded deoxiribonucleic acid (DNA) with LTR. The newly produced retroviral DNA is still associated with some viral enzymes and core proteins; together they form the pre-integration complex. FIV possesses the capacity to infect both non-dividing and dividing cells. In the latter, the pre-integration complex can access the host DNA easily during mitosis. For infection of non-replicating cells, active transport of the pre-integration complex in the cellular nucleus is necessary. A polypurine tract located centrally in the FIV genome and designated as central DNA flap has been held responsible for this function [32]. The viral IN catalyzes the integration of viral DNA in the host's cell DNA. Interestingly, the integration of the virus does not take place at a specific site in the host genome, but rather occurs randomly at different sites.

Integrated viral DNA, called provirus, behaves very much like a eukaryotic gene. It may be transcribed into full-length transcripts using host cell RNA Polymerase II in order to produce more virus, or it may remain latent for long periods of time and replicate when cellular DNA is replicated by the cell. Each infected cell thus transmits the viral genome to its descendants.

For the efficient production of new virus particles, the full-length transcripts follow three different routes. Some are exported from the nucleus and serve as mRNA for viral *gag* and *pol* protein precursors, which are translated by cytoplasmic ribosomes. Other full-length RNA molecules are spliced directly in the nucleus to form mRNA for the *env* protein precursors. *env* mRNA is translated by ribosomes bound to the endoplasmatic reticulum, and thereby produced proteins are glycosylated in the Golgi apparatus and cleaved by cellular proteases to form the mature TM-SU complex. These mature proteins are then delivered to the surface of the cell. Finally, other full-length transcripts are transported into the cytoplasm and serve directly as progeny viral genomes.

All viral parts produced in this way assemble at budding sites at the inner surface of the plasma membrane. During budding, the virus receives its envelope, consisting of parts of the cell membrane and viral glycoproteins. Simultaneously, the virally encoded PR, which is itself a component of the core precursor protein, cleaves at specific sites within *gag* and *pol* precursors to produce mature, infectious viral particles, now free to infect new target cells in the host. The main steps of FIV replication are summarized in figure 3.

Literature

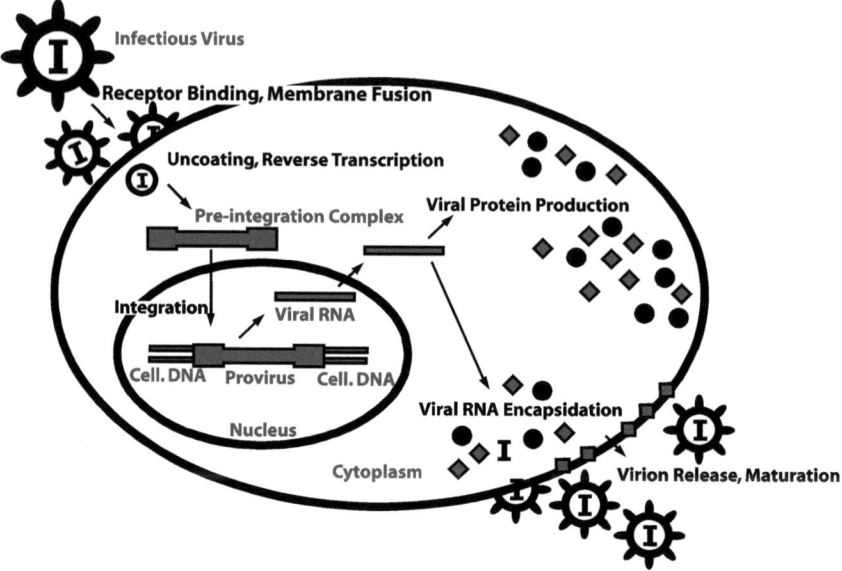

Figure 3: Main steps of the FIV replication cycle

3.1.3 Pathogenesis

3.1.3.1 Viral transmission

FIV can be isolated from blood, serum, plasma, cerebrospinal fluid and saliva of experimentally or naturally infected cats by cell or tissue culture methods [25, 33].

In field conditions, shedding in saliva is most relevant, and aggressive biting is considered the most important route of transmission. Indeed, older, free-roaming male cats are more prone to infection due to exhibition of territorial behaviour. In addition, cats living in environments with high population density belong to high risk groups, although the virus is not efficiently spread by casual non-aggressive contact between cats. When kept strictly indoors, cats rarely become infected and a low prevalence in breeding cats is predominantly due to the fact that they are mostly kept under restricted living conditions.

FIV is present in semen of naturally and experimentally infected cats [34], and veneral transmission seems possible. Artificial insemination performed with fresh semen from experimentally infected cats effectively infected FIV-naïve queens in 50% of the cases [35]. Transmission of FIV by mating however remains relevant under field conditions mainly due to the fact that male cats most often bite the queens during mating.

Of particular interest is the possibility of vertical transmission resulting in productive infection and disease in offspring. FIV-infected mothers in phases of high viral load (see 3.1.3.2) can effectively transmit the virus to their kittens. Transplacental transmission of FIV to the kittens occurred in 2/3 cases after either intravenous or subcutaneous infection of the queen three weeks prior to parturition [36]. Moreover, mothers inoculated with FIV immediately post-partum can infect newborn kittens via milk [37]. Interestingly, more recent studies show that the frequency of perinatal FIV transmission from infected queens to their kittens seems to correlate with chronicity of infection and maternal symptoms of clinical immunodeficiency [38].

In experimental studies, transmission via mucosal and parenteral (intravenous, intraperitoneal, subcutaneous) routes have proven to be efficient. Virus strains representing at least three clades of FIV can be transmitted across the vaginal, rectal, or oral mucosa [39]. However, up to 10^4 fold more virus is required for infection by mucosal routes in comparison to parenteral routes [40].

3.1.3.2 Course of Disease

The kinetics of FIV infection vary according to virus isolate and route of exposure. The following refers to a general pattern of infection, which can be approximately extrapolated to the various forms of FIV disease.

The course of FIV infection is divided into five clinically recognizable phases, which naturally correlate with pathogenetic progression of disease: 1) acute infection, 2) asymptomatic phase, 3) persistent generalized lymphadenopathy, 4) AIDS-related complex (ARC), and 5) AIDS phase. The clinical aspects of theses stages are described in more detail under 3.1.5.

FIV infection is characterized by progressive immune deterioration. Hallmarks of disease progression include CD4+ lymphocyte counts in blood and CD4+:CD8+ lymphocyte ratio [41], specific cytotoxic lymphocyte (CTL) counts, antibody titers as well as proviral load in PBMCs [42] and viral load in plasma [43] (figure 4).

Lymphoctyes of CD4+ phenotype are primary targets of infection. Additionally, a significant infection of macrophages takes place already during the acute phase of the disease. Proviral DNA can thus be detected in PBMCs as early as five days after infection, and infectious virus can be isolated from lymphocytes as of day 10 post-infection. Viremia then rapidly increases until week 3, peaks between weeks 7 and 8 and then decreases again during the asymptomatic phase of disease. In the terminal stage, virus replicates again efficiently and viral load increases accordingly in plasma. When virus peaks in the acute phase of infection, CD4+ cells decrease by approximately one third due to primary viral replication in these cells. However, a slow rise can be observed as the severity of viremia decreases. During the asymptomatic phase, CD4+ cells decrease only very slowly, while a very rapid decrease occurs together with the terminal AIDS stage of disease. As early as two weeks after the onset of infection, the CD8+ lymphocyte population expands rapidly. The antiviral activity of this population subset induces reduction of viremia. During the asymptomatic phase of disease, the total CD8+ lymphocyte count tends to remain at a rate higher than normal, and decreases again to very low counts in terminal stages of disease.

Antibodies against FIV have been detected in experimentally and naturally infected cats as early as 2-3 weeks following infection and persist throughout the different phases of disease. High antibody levels correlate with the viremia peak in the acute phase of infection.

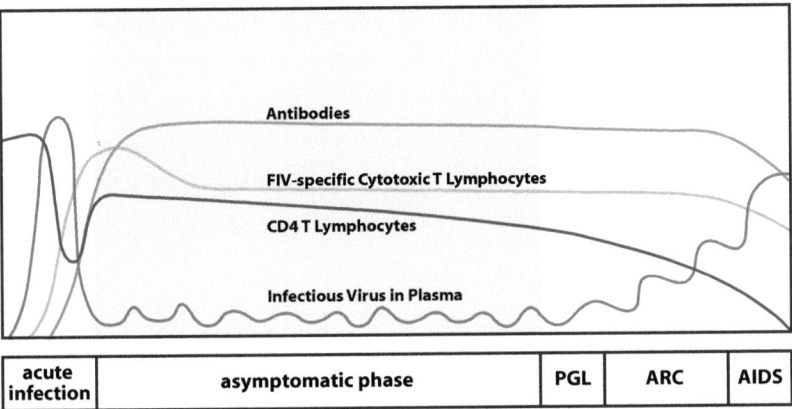

Figure 4: Graphical representation of the course of viremia, antibody production, circulating CD4+ and specific cytotoxic lymphocytes in the blood of infected cats during the different stages of infection.

3.1.3.3 Immunological Aspects

The pathogenesis of FIV is to date not completely understood. Infected cats develop latency despite elaboration of defence mechanisms such as specific cellular immune responses and production of neutralizing antibodies.

This chapter represents an overview of the important known immunological processes during FIV infection of the domestic cat.

3.1.3.3.1 CD4+ T Lymphocyte Depletion

All FIV isolates and all routes of infection commonly lead to a decline of CD4+ lymphocyte count in the peripheral blood of the infected cat. AIDS stage of disease is often defined by a concentration of less than 200 CD4+ T cells/µl whole blood, although CD4+ cytopenia is clearly not responsible alone for terminal stage immune dysfunction.

Decrease in CD4+ cells depends on several mechanisms but is usually due to a reduced life span of the cells. The quantitative decrease, however, cannot just be explained by cytolysis as a result of viral infection, because the percentage of infected cells is significantly lower than the number of cells dying. As a consequence, FIV-mediated T cell depletion and lymphocyte activation have been related to an accelerated cell death or apoptosis and it has been shown that lymphocytes from FIV-infected cats are prone to die after short term culture *in vitro* [44]. Additionally, the extent of *in vitro* lymphocyte apoptosis was shown to correlate with progression of disease [45]. More recent and detailed information on T cell depletion and apoptosis is discussed under 3.1.3.3.3.

3.1.3.3.2 CD8+ T Lymphocyte Antiviral Activity

Rapid expansion of the CD8+ lymphocyte subset, along with specific anti-FIV cytolytic and non-cytolytic mechanisms, arise early in the course of FIV infection, even before a noticeable humoral immune response. Appearance of this antiviral activity corresponds to a reduction in viremia and transition to the asymptomatic stage of disease [46]. Interestingly, although CTL responses against *gag* and *env* antigens have been described, persistent high-level circulating antiviral CTL could not be detected during FIV infection, as has been observed in HIV-infected humans [47]. CTL responses seem to become localized in the lymph nodes and spleen with progression of disease [48]. Non-cytolytic CD8+ lymphocyte responses are detectable earlier than cytotoxic mechanisms. Also, since non-cytolytic processes are not MHC-restricted, they have a more diverse action potential. The inhibitory effect is mediated by soluble factors and, as a consequence, is not dependent on direct cell-to-cell contact [49]. Further studies allowed to more precisely allot this CD8+ T cell anti-FIV activity at the level of FIV mRNA synthesis from the FIV proviral DNA [50]. Moreover, acute stage of FIV infection is characterized by the appearance of a CD8+ T cell subpopulation showing reduced expression of the CD8 β chain and complete disappearance of the L-selectin CD62L surface molecule [51]. These CD8βlowCD62L T cells then persist throughout the course of infection, and recent studies have demonstrated that a subset of T cells, the TNFα+CD8+ T cells, that specifically respond to FIV antigens in the course of infection by production of tumor necrosis factor α (TNFα), are contained in this CD8βlowCD62L T cell subpopulation [52].

3.1.3.3.3 T Cell Dysfunction, Anergy and Apoptosis

Already in the acute phase of infection, defects in T cell responses are encountered. Mitogen and antigen induced IL-2 production and lymphoproliferation are reduced in the acute phase and continue to decline with progression of disease [41].

The B7.1 and B7.2 co-stimulatory molecules on antigen-presenting cells provide second signals for regulating T cell immune responses via CD28 and CTL antigen 4 (CTLA4) on T cells. CD28 signals cell proliferation, whereas CTLA4 signals for anergy or apoptosis, terminating the immune response. Flow cytometry revealed high percentages of CD8+ and CD4+ cells expressing B7.1, B7.2, and CTLA4 in lymph nodes of FIV-NCSU1-positive cats and a large fraction of CTLA4+ T cells co-expressing B7.1 and B7.2 [53]. Moreover, anti-B7.1 antibodies significantly inhibited T cell apoptosis in FIV-infected cats with low level plasma viremia, further suggesting that lymph node apoptosis and immune deterioration in FIV-infected cats may result from chronic B7-CTLA4-mediated T-T negative signalling interactions [54].

Further understanding of mechanisms for T cell depletion and dysfunction comes from studies of regulatory T cells (Treg). CD4+ regulatory cells prevent the activation of autoreactive T cells, and help to maintain self-tolerance. Detection of CD25 (the IL-2 receptor alpha chain) has been used to identify the subpopulation of CD4+ T cells which have regulatory function. CD25+ subsets of CD4+ as well as CD8+ T cells increase in lymph node of FIV-NCSU1 infected cats very early after exposure to the virus. The CD4+CTLA4+B7+ phenotype described in FIV-positive cats interestingly resembles the CD4+CD25+CTLA4+ phenotype described for immunosuppressive Treg cells. Additionally, similar to Treg cells, feline CD4+CD25+ T cells directly isolated from lymph nodes of FIV-infected cats do not produce IL-2, fail to proliferate in response to mitogen stimulation, and suppress the proliferative response and the IL-2 production of Concanavalin A (Con A)-stimulated autologous CD4+CD25- T cells. These FIV-negative, activated, anergic, immunosuppressive CD25+CTLA4+B7+CD4+ Treg-like cells may contribute to the progressive loss of T cell immune function that is typical of FIV infection [55].

Further characterization of these T cell subpopulations indicate possible mechanisms of FIV latency, typically encountered during FIV infection. While both CD4+CD25+ and CD4+CD25- cells are susceptible to FIV infection *in vitro* and *in vivo*, only CD4+CD25+ cells produce infectious virions when cultured with IL-2. Latently infected CD4+CD25- cells produce infectious virions only following ConA stimulation. Furthermore, CD4+CD25+ cells remain relatively resistant to apoptosis, independent of their infection with FIV. Altogether, these findings define CD4+CD25+ cells as main characters for productive FIV infection. CD4+CD25- cells however, represent a potential latent viral reservoir capable of being reactivated after stimulation [56].

3.1.3.3.4 Cytokine Production

Dysregulation in cytokine expression has been well described in acute and chronic FIV infection. In FIV-infected cats, CD4+ lymphocytes produce TNF-α, Interferon (INF)-γ, Interkeukin (IL)-2, IL-4, and IL-10, while CD8+ lymphocytes express TNF-α, INF-γ and IL-2. Monocytes and macrophages are the source of IL-1, IL-6, TNF-α, IL-10 and IL-12 [57]. Whole blood and relevant lymphoid tissues such as lymph nodes, spleen and thymus demonstrate unique cytokine profiles that differ qualitatively and quantitatively during infection, and correlate with virus replication in each tissue or organ [58].

Serum levels of IL-1, IL-6, TNF-α and IFN-γ are increased with FIV infection and are higher in symptomatic versus asymptomatic cats [59].

It is well established that cytokines such as IFN-γ and TNF-α, produced by T cells upon antigen stimulation, are important for controlling viral infections. Increasing TNF-α levels during the acute phase of infection are associated with virus replication [60]. It has now also been demonstrated, that FIV-infected cats develop both IFN-γ+ and TNF-α+ FIV-specific T cell subpopulations early in the course of infection [52].

IFN-γ, also called type II IFN, is produced by activated T cells and natural killer (NK) cells and is known for its immunomodulatory and antiviral activities. Surprisingly, in contrast to feline type I IFN, which have been reported to inhibit *in vitro* replication of FIV as well as other common feline viruses, feline INF-γ seemingly lacks potential to inhibit infection of PBMCs [61]. These results suggest that the main function of IFN-γ produced during infection may not be the direct inhibition of FIV replication. Instead, indirect effects of IFN-γ such as increase of cytotoxic T cell and NK cell responses to virus-infected cells may play a more central role in controlling the infection. Nevertheless, it is accepted that presence of IFN-γ production during FIV infection reflects a functional immune system, whereas the loss of IFN-γ production correlates with progression to AIDS.

TNF-α production plays an important role in the pathogenesis of FIV. Production of this cytokine correlates with appearance of virus in plasma and tissues [60]. Moreover, TNF-α is apparently associated with an increased apoptosis susceptibility of FIV- infected cells and might be involved in FIV-specific T cell depletion [62]. Whether TNF-α production by FIV-specific T cells is beneficial or detrimental for FIV-infected cats still needs to be determined.

IL-1 and IL-6 are cytokines generally produced in the course of infectious processes. In addition to pro-inflammatory effects, the elevated production of IL-6 may contribute to polyclonal B cell activation and gammopathies [63].

Peak production of IL-1, IL-6 and TNF during FIV infection coincided with periods of depressed immune responses *in vivo* and the presence of clinical signs. Additionally, high expression of these pro-inflammotory cytokines concurs with depressed responsiveness of PBMCs to mitogenic stimulation *in vitro* [59].

Dysregulation of cytokine responses in FIV-infected versus FIV-naïve cats induces inability to effectively fight against secondary pathogens. Observed cytokine profile during secondary opportunistic infections with *Toxoplasma gondii* [64] or *Listeria monocytogenes* [65] indicate a loss of the important T helper (Th) 1 cellular immune response during FIV infection.

Although controversed for a long time, it is now overall accepted that the cytokine patterns seen in the course of FIV infection implicate a dominating Th2 type immune response, and that attempts to elaborate effective vaccines should concentrate on supporting and enhancing Th1-orientated T helper responses.

3.1.3.3.5 Antibody Responses

FIV-infected cats develop a strong immune response against the viral *gag* and *env* proteins. Moreover, parts of the SU, the TM and *gag* proteins are considered major B cell epitopes. Cats infected experimentally can seroconvert already 2-3 weeks post-challenge, and antibodies against envelope proteins seem to arise first, followed by a response against *gag* elements [66].

Antigen stimulation of infected B cells is increased compared to non-infected cells, and a polyclonal gammopathy directed against non-viral proteins may be seen in FIV-infected cats as early as 6 weeks post infection [63].

The development of virus-neutralizing antibodies (VN) during many viral infections is one of the most effective host defence mechanisms. Interestingly, FIV infection *in vivo* persists in spite of the production of high VN titres. The V3-V5 areas of the *env* gene are known to code for neutralizing epitopes of FIV. It has been shown that single amino acid substitution mutations in the envelope glycoprotein, within or outside the VN epitopes, may confer resistance to monoclonal or polyclonal VN [67]. *In vitro* sensitive FIV strains have shown reversion to neutralization resistance due to mutations in V4 and V5 regions of the *env* gene, after passage *in vivo* for 4-15 months. This mutated phenotype appears to be essential for survival and persistence of virus *in vivo* [68].

A long term study following experimentally infected cats has indicated a progressive increase in VN titres during the first 30 weeks post-inoculation, followed by stably high titres for an observation period of 7 years thereafter [69]. Cross-clade neutralization is common [70], indicating that important neutralization-inducing epitopes are universally shared in spite of the high antigenic diversity in FIV strains prevailing in the field.

3.1.4 Epidemology

3.1.4.1 Viral Clades

FIV is endemic in cats throughout the world. Five distinct clades of FIV (A-E) have been identified based on greater than 15-30 % variability in envelope amino acid sequence. The majority of viruses identified to date belong to either clade A or clade B. The prototype virus, FIV-Petaluma, discovered in 1986 by Pedersen and colleagues, is attributed to clade A, a group of strains significantly less diverse than clade B, and containing fewer genomic mutations, suggesting more recent, less host-adapted strains [71]. Clade A viruses are present worldwide with a predominance in the western United States, northern Japan, Germany, and South Africa. Also distributed worldwide, clade B viruses have been more consistently identified in eastern Japan, Italy, Portugal, and the central and eastern United States. With the exception of northern Taiwan, detection of clade C FIV remains uncommon, and has often only been attributed to single animals or small groups of cats from Vancouver, Munich and Japan [72]. Clade D includes several viruses characterized mainly in western Japan [73]. Finally, two Argentinian strains comprise clade E [74].

Similarly to other lentiviruses, FIV is very susceptible to evolutionary genetic alterations and, as a consequence, phenotypic variability. Genetic diversity both due to evolution of the virus within an infected individual and to recombination following dual infection have been described for FIV. Indeed, intra-individual *env* variation is known to be the major determinant of viral diversity in virus isolates [75]. Recent studies have however demonstrated stable maintenance of the V3-V5 *env* gene encoding neutralizing epitopes for 1-2 years after infection [76]. Co-infection with two strains, although uncommon, has been successfully established under experimental conditions [77] and its occurrence confirmed in naturally infected animals [71]. It has also been demonstrated that biological behaviour and pathogenicity differ from one isolate to another [78]. Thus, properties identified for a specific strain cannot be generalized, and regular phylogenetic studies allowing evaluation of evolutionary viral adaptation to the host are a prerequisite when developing new treatments or prophylactic measures.

Literature

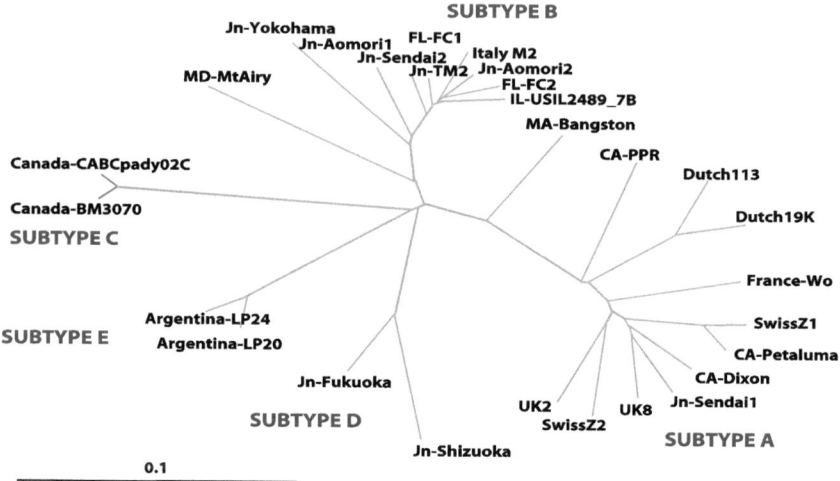

Figure 5: The phylogenetic tree distinction of the main known FIV subtypes and strains. Isolates from Japan JN and isolates from the USA are designated with the state abbreviation followed by the name of the virus. The scale indicates 1% difference in envelope sequences. Adapted from [197].

3.1.4.2 Host Range

Domestic cats (*felis catus*) are the natural hosts for FIV. However, cross-reactive antibodies have been detected in over half of the species of the family Felidae [79]. Transmission of FIV from domestic to non-domestic cats has been reported [80], but the majority of FIV-reactive antibodies in non-domestic cats are induced by other FIV-related species-specific lentiviruses, as described for the puma, *Puma concolor* [81], the lion, *Panthera leo* [82], and the Pallas' cat, *Otocolobus manul* [83]. These viruses are known to be older and more stable than FIV, and recent studies surprisingly indicate that they diverge greatly in amino acid sequences, host cell susceptibility, receptor affinity, neutralizing antibody binding sites, and pathogenicity, when compared to FIV [84]. Non-domestic cat lentiviruses can also establish persistent infection in domestic cats, however clinical disease is frequently absent [85]. Interestingly, infection of domestic cats with a non-domestic lentivirus generates humoral and cell-mediated immune responses and thus provides partial protection from disease induced by superinfection with FIV [86].

Infection of human cell lines with FIV result in proviral integration [29] and at least two FIV strains have been able to infect human PBMCs and macrophages *in vitro* [30]. Moreover, experimental FIV infection of cynomolgus macaques resulted in loss of CD4+ cells and weight loss [87]. Cross packaging of HIV-1, SIV and FIV RNA have been demonstrated, suggesting that co-infection could result in stable recombinant viruses [88]. However, these findings must be considered with precaution, and should not be extrapolated to suggesting that infection of human beings with FIV can occur. Replication of FIV has to date not been observed in human cells, and lack of human seroreactivity despite significant exposure to infected cats indicate very low potential for zoonosis among healthy adult humans [89].

3.1.4.3 Occurrence and Prevalence Studies

Several seroepidemiological surveys have revealed an overall seroprevalence worldwide of 11,04 % among both healthy and sick cats screened in North America, Asia, Europe and Oceania [90]. It is important to keep in mind that prevalence rates vary greatly by region, lifestyle, health status and gender of the cats tested. Furthermore, these studies are likely to underestimate reality, since they often fail to take into consideration that a considerable portion of FIV-infected cats are seronegative (see also 3.1.6). Table 2 represents the more recent prevalence studies carried out on different continents.

Literature

Continent	Country	Prevalence (%)	Reference
Europe			
	Switzerland	0.7-3.4	91
	Norway	5.9 - 10.1	92
	France	22.0	93
	Great Britain	6.0 - 19.0	94-96
	Italy	12.5 - 24.0	97, 98
	Germany	2.0 - 3.0	99
	Spain	8.3	100
	Czech Republic	5.8	101
	Turkey (Istanbul)	22.3	102
America			
	USA	10.2 - 15.2	103, 104
	Canada / USA	1.2 - 14.0	104
Asia			
	Japan	9.8	105
	Taiwan	4.0	106
	Vietnam	22.0	107
Oceania			
	Australia	13.5 -32.0	108, 109
	New Zealand	37.0	110

Table 2: Relevant FIV prevalence studies carried out on the different continents

3.1.5 Clinical Aspects

Similarly to HIV infection in humans, FIV causes progressive immune deterioration in domestic cats. Since individuals become persistently infected, complete recovery is not possible, and infected cats eventually die of the disease. Although all categories of domestic cats may become infected, susceptibility to FIV infection and disease progression are inversely related to age [111]. The clinical progression of FIV can be defined in five stages, using the system described for HIV infection in humans [112]: 1) acute infection, 2) asymptomatic phase, 3) persistent generalized lymphadenopathy, 4) AIDS-related complex (ARC), and 5) AIDS phase. Distinct clinical features for these stages are summarized in table 3.

During the acute phase of infection, the cat usually shows only little or no

Stage	Clinical Signs	Duration
Acute Infection	apathy, lymphadenopathy, fever	weeks to months
Asymptomatic Phase	no clinical signs	months to years
Persistent Generalized Lymphadenopathy	generalized lymphadenopathy	weeks to months
AIDS-related complex	recurrent fever, apathy, anorexia, weight loss chronic stomatitis, behavioral abnormalities	several months to 1 year
AIDS Phase	symptoms of AIDS-related complex opportunistc infections, neoplasia	Several months

Table 3: Main clinical symptoms of the different stages of FIV infection

symptoms at all. Typical are low-grade fever and generalized lymphadenopathy eventually accompanied by slight lethargy [113]. Unfortunately, owners often fail to notice these rather mild and unspecific signs, and clinical suspicion of disease is only assessed after greater progression of the infection. Characterization of clincal lymphadenopathy in FIV-infected cats has revealed histopathological alterations in the lymph nodes of the hindlimb, forelimb and head, in decreasing order of severity, with little evidence of involvement of the alimentary tract-associated lymph nodes [114]. The popliteal lymph node is thus considered a good indicator for assessment of lymph node status in FIV infection.

The clinical signs of the ARC and AIDS stages are diverse in nature because symptoms due to primary viral infection are frequently overlapped by those of an array of secondary infections [115]. Slow but progressive weight loss is common, with severe wasting occurring late in the disease process. Fever of 40°C or greater is often present. Loss of appetite or evidence of pain while eating, caused by gingivitis and stomatitis, are also typical. Chronic, non-responsive, or recurrent infections of the skin, alimentary tract, upper respiratory tract and eyes are often observed [104]. Infection may lead to abortion of kittens or other reproductive failures in pregnant queens [116]. Encephalopathy-linked neurological abnormalities, although rather rare, mostly induce behavioural alterations. However, dementia, twitching movements of the face and tongue, loss of bladder and rectal control, cognitive and behavioural alterations and compulsive roaming have all been recognized in FIV-infected cats. Seizures, ataxia and intentions tremor have also been described [117]. Renal involvement in FIV disease has been described as a frequent occurrence and direct consequence of viral infection. Moreover, presence of immuncomplexes in renal tissue suggest that immunological processes in the course of FIV infection play a role in the pathogenesis of renal damage [118]. Interestingly, no link has been established between FIV infection and lower urinary tract disease, a relatively common disorder in adult cats [119].

The role of FIV in tumorigenesis is still quite controversial. As reported for SIV and HIV, it has been postulated that occurrence of lymphoma could be related to infection in FIV seropositive cats. [120]. The majority of presumed FIV-associated lymphomas are of B cell blastic phenotype and usually occur at a single extranodal site [121]. Examination for FIV provirus in tumorous cells has however been inconsistent in both experimentally and naturally infected cats, and the amount of cases remains small. Lymphoid malignancies, myeloproliferative diseases, and several carcinomas and sarcomas have also been more frequently detected in FIV-infected, feline leukaemia virus (FeLV)-naïve cats, suggesting a potential association between FIV and malignancy.

Secondary infection during ARC and AIDS stages of disease can be due to various microorganisms which take advantage of the weakened immune system, including other viruses, bacteria, parasites and fungi. The most commonly detected opportunistic microorganisms detected in the course of FIV infections are summarized in table 4.

Among predisposition to other parasitical infections related to FIV disease, toxoplasmosis, as an opportunistic infection in HIV-infected humans, is of high interest. Primary infection of cats with FIV markedly enhance their susceptibility to a secondary *Toxoplasma gondii* infection [122]. Furthermore, FIV-infected cats develop higher *T.gondii* IgM antibody levels and show increased replication rate of *T.gondii* [123].

Another frequently studied association is that of FIV and FeLV infections. Seroepidemiologic surveys have indicated that dual infection is not uncommon, and that cats infected with both viruses tend to have a more severe disease course and die sooner than mono-infected animals [124]. Moreover, FeLV infection has proven to enhance FIV infection *in vitro* and *in vivo* by facilitating expression and spread of FIV in the body, leading to faster decline of the immune system and earlier signs of infection [113].

Certain changes in blood and bone marrow parameters are consistently observed in FIV-infected animals. In the primary stage, a leucopenia, associated initially with a mild lymphopenia and later by both a mild lymphopenia and a severe neutropenia, is frequently observed [33, 125]. Towards the end of the disease, in ARC and AIDS stages, common findings include anemia, lymphopenia, thrombocytopenia, neutropenia in blood, as well as hyperplasia of individual cell lineages and dismorphic alterations in bone marrow [126]. In addition, several significant alterations in clinical chemistry have been noted as of the ninth month post-infection: divergences in glucose, protein, gamma globulin, sodium, urea, phosphorus, lipase, cholesterol, and triglyceride levels in serum have been described [127]. However, these abnormalities are not pathognomonic for FIV infection and are therefore not reliable in characterization of disease progression. Markers representing more effectively the impairment of the immune system and allowing prediction of clinical outcome are CD4+:CD8+ lymphocyte ratio and plasma viral load [128].

Literature

Type of Infection	Pathogen	Reference
Viral	Feline Leukemia Virus (FeLV)	95, 104, 124, 129, 130
	Feline Calicivirus (FCV)	131-133
	Feline Herpes Virus (FHV)	134
	Feline Coronavirus (FCoV)	129
	Feline Papillomavirus	135
	Pox Virus	136
Bacterial	Streptococcus Canis	137
	Mycobacteria	110, 129, 138
Protozoal	Toxoplasma	122, 123, 129, 139, 140
	Cryptosporidia	141
	Hemobartonella	103, 129, 142
Parasital	Demodex Cati	110, 113
	Notoedres	113, 129
Fungal	Candida Albicans	129, 138
	Cryptococcus	129, 138, 143

Table 4: Most common opportunistic pathogens observed in the context of FIV infection

3.1.6 Diagnostic Approach

In addition to multiple haematological, serum biological and cytological bone marrow abnormalities which may lead to suspicion of an FIV infection, several elaborated laboratory tests allow confirmation of the diagnosis. The various tools developed over time since discovery of the virus are briefly described below.

Enzyme-linked immunosorbent assay (ELISA) tests are available in kit form for use in private veterinary clinics, and are usually used as screening tests. One variant, which detects antibodies against the FIV TM and *gag* proteins, is commercially available. Since cats do not recover from FIV, detection of antibodies in the serum can be directly correlated with presence of FIV infection. Antibodies to FIV can be detected as early as 30 days after exposure, and during the rest of the infected animal's life. Clinical signs can however appear before seroconversion and some cats show no detectable levels of antibodies in their blood for many weeks [144]. Moreover, antibody levels can fall below detection level in the final stage of disease [104]. Altogether, these facts can lead to occurrence of false negative reactions. In addition, the specificity of ELISA tests is unfortunately not optimal. Positive results should always be considered in relation to prevalence, and confirmed by a second test in healthy or low-risk cats [145]. Confirmatory tests, performed commonly at diagnostic laboratories, include Western Blot or Indirect Fluorescent Antibody Immunoassays (IFAI).

The major advantage of Western Blot immunoassays is the detection, in one reaction, of antibodies against various viral proteins. Methods were described rapidly after discovery of FIV [146, 147]. A densitometric analysis of Western Blots enabling to quantify the antibodies against FIV proteins has also been described [148].

In turn, detection of antibodies by IFAI is based on the binding of specific antibodies in diluted serum samples to antigen expressed by FIV-infected T lymphocyte enriched PBMCs or CRFK cells as substrate. In a second step, bound antibodies are stained with fluorescein labelled anti-cat antibodies and made visible with the fluorescence microscope [149].

It is worthwhile mentioning here that kittens can have detectable colostrum-derived antibodies for several months. Therefore, only kittens older than 6 months with positive results in both ELISA and confirmatory tests can be considered infected.

ELISA tests detecting antibodies of various specificities have been elaborated over the years. It has been demonstrated that over 90 percent of FIV-infected cats establish an antibody response to the reverse transcriptase enzyme. This response displays increasing *in vitro* inhibitory effects over time post-infection. Unfortunately, significant concentrations of reverse transcriptase inhibiting antibodies are detected only 1 to 2 years after infection, rendering their detection rather irrelevant in routine diagnostics [150]. In 1992, Furuya and co-workers developed an ELISA system for detection of antibodies to FIV *gag* protein in cat sera [151]. They thereby observed increases of the antibody titers to FIV *gag* protein in all studied cases, already at an early stage of infection. However, the establishment of ELISA systems using recombinant SU, TM and CA antigens of FIV and comparison of their individual efficiency showed highest diagnostic sensitivity (98%), accompanied by a specificity of 97 % in the case of detection of TM antibodies. Furthermore, antibodies to TM appeared first after infection rendering this antigen most important for diagnostic purposes [152].

Detection of a FIV antigen in infected cats is of low interest in routine diagnostics due to the often insignificant levels of virus in plasma during the asymptomatic phase of disease. Moreover, although the establishment of a p24 antigen capture ELISA system for research purposes has shown convincing potential for monitoring FIV replication *in vitro* [153], p24 *in vivo* is commonly decorated with antibodies and therefore not reliably detectable.

Various cell culture techniques have also been established to identify cellular or plasma-related viremia. Thus, isolation and *in vitro* stimulation of PBMCs with subsequent detection of produced viral antigen allows the assessment of cellular infection. With the intention to simplify such experiments, Guiot and co-workers developed an assay allowing direct culture of small amounts of whole blood (100 µl), followed by detection of FIV core *gag* antigen released in culture supernatants [154]. Avoiding the hassle of leukocyte separation and lymphocyte purification procedures, this technique offers many advantages and shows convincing reproducibility. Moreover, several FIV-sensitive cell lines allow the assessment of infectious virus in plasma of infected cats (see 3.1.2.2). A T lymphoblastoid cell line obtained from the PBMCs of a spf cat and designated MBM was even reported to exhibit a lytic cytopathic effect *in vitro* upon FIV infection [28].

The development of polymerase chain reaction (PCR) assays represents a significant step for the identification of the proviral and viral forms of FIV in routine diagnostics, as a complement to common methods, as well as in research areas. Detection of provirus by a nested PCR method using regions of the *gag* gene as target sequences was described as early as 1992 [155, 156]. Soon after, Matteucci and colleagues established an assay allowing detection of FIV RNA [157]. Although sophisticated and complex, these early PCR methods often failed to harbour satisfying sensitivity levels. The need in further understanding of pathogenesis and pressure in the development of new markers of disease progression induced establishment of quantitative PCR methods. In this way, Inoshima and colleagues described an assay for the measurements of proviral DNA copies in Japanese strains [158]. Furthermore, using *in vitro* synthesized RNA derived from the *gag* region of the FIV genome as competitive control, Vahlenkamp et al. succeeded in quantifying FIV RNA from plasma of infected cats [159].

The latest evolution in quantification of FIV DNA and RNA is the TaqMan fluorogenic real-time detection system [160]. This improved PCR method is based on the 5'-3' exonuclease activity of the Taq DNA polymerase, which results in cleavage of a fluorescent dye labelled probe during the amplification cycles. The intensity of fluorescence is then measured by a Sequence Detection System. A more detailed characterization of the TaqMan system is described in section 4.2.3.

Further characterization of FIV pathogenesis *in vivo* relies on the localization of virus to specific cells in tissues, enabling detection of host-virus interactions at different time points in disease. FIV was most often revealed in tissue sections by *in situ* RNA hybridization. Unfortunately, tissue digestion steps required for *in situ* RNA hybridization often destroy protease sensitive cell specific antigens, limiting the number of protein markers available to identify the cells infected. Identification of FIV-specific proteins by immunohistochemistry circumvents the need for protease digestion steps and RNase free protocols. However, both conventionally used mouse monoclonal and rabbit polyclonal antibodies lack specificity and sensitivity in binding FIV in tissue sections. In 2002, Rogers and colleagues established an immunohistochemical protocol using high antibody titer serum from cats chronically infected with FIV-PET [161]. This method includes labeling of native species antibodies with horse-radish peroxidase (HRP) before their binding on tissues. Presence of FIV in the tissue can then be detected by standard chromogenic or fluorescence techniques. In complement to other *in situ* methodologies, this assay allows quantitation of virus in tissues from cats infected with either FIV clade B or clade C. Such steps in diagnostic research contribute to the further understanding of important processes concerning tropism and replication kinetics of FIV infection *in vivo*.

Literature

3.1.7 Treatment

Unfortunately, there is to date no treatment allowing effective elimination of FIV in an infected cat. As a consequence, therapy of FIV-associated disease is mostly supportive, with the objective of increasing the patient's life quality and length. In addition to treatments such as antiviral and immune stimulation drugs, immunodeficient cats in the late stages of disease may require appropriate long term antimicrobial therapy or multiple treatment periods to fight secondary opportunistic infections.

Various approaches in treatment against FIV have been evaluated. Over the years, researchers have been greatly inspired by the progress in treatment of HIV. Indeed, the most promising results to date include drugs interfering directly with retroviral replication, derived from HIV research.

Four classes of antiretroviral agents are currently available for the treatment of HIV infection: nucleoside and nucleotide analogs, also referred to as reverse transcriptase inhibitors (NRTIs), non-nucleoside reverse transcriptase inhibitors (NNRTIs), protease inhibitors (PIs) and fusion inhibitors. The highly active antiretroviral therapy (HAART), commonly administered to HIV-infected patients, consists of a combination of three drugs from one or more of the above mentioned groups. Typically, the therapy includes one NRTI, one PI and either a second NRTI or a NNRTI. The major problem encountered during antiretroviral therapy is the appearance of resistance to treatment due to mutative adaptation of the virus. Chronically HIV-infected patients having received various combinations of HAART over several years may develop multi-resistant strains of the virus, rendering treatment ineffective. As a consequence, although a wide range of drugs exist, there is a constant need for new therapeutic strategies.

Treatment effectiveness of all four classes of antiretroviral agents and in various combinations has been experimented for FIV.

The direct target of NRTIs is the retroviral enzyme reverse transcriptase. Acting as alternative substrates, they compete with physiological nucleosides, differing from them only by a minor modification in their ribose molecule. The incorporation of nucleoside analogs aborts DNA synthesis by the RT, as phosphodiester bridges can no longer be built to stabilize the double strand. NRTIs are not HIV-specific inhibitors as they are broadly effective to other lentiviruses as well, including FIV [162]. Azidothymidine (AZT), a thymidine analog also designated zidovudine, was the first antiretroviral agent to be put on the market for HIV treatment. Early studies still tested AZT as monotherapy. In 1993, Meers and colleagues described a significant reduction of plasma virus titre by zidovudine treatments in asymptomatic FIV-infected cats, begun 24 hours post-infection and continued for 4 weeks [163]. The FIV titres in PBMCs however, were high for the whole duration of the experiment. Furthermore, in a study evaluating long term effectiveness of AZT compared with conventional symptomatical therapy in FIV-seropositive diseased cats, AZT led to total recovery from clinical symptoms in six of nine FIV-seropositive cats 4-6 weeks after the onset of therapy. Although all the FIV-seropositive cats treated symptomatically in this study responded well to antibiotics and immunomodulators within as little as 10 to 14 days, recurrence of severe clinical symptoms was noticed in most cases [164].

In the interest of diminishing undesired adverse effects of AZT monotherapy such as anemia and hypoproteinemia, researchers have more recently tested the reliability of NRTI combinations. Lamivudine (3TC), is a well tolerated cytosine analog in clinical use against HIV. *In vitro* studies utilizing AZT alone, lamivudine (3TC) alone, or AZT/3TC combination against FIV indicated that simultaneous treatments of AZT and 3TC generated additive to synergistic effects in primary PBMCs, but not in chronically infected cell lines. Similarly, AZT/3TC combination induced a significant delay in infection and seroconversion in unprotected cats, but had no anti-FIV activity in chronically infected cats. AZT/3TC treatment seems therefore effective for prophylaxis but not for therapeutic use in chronically FIV-infected cats [165]. An alternative to 3TC is stampidine, the latest nucleoside analog prepared for treatment of HIV. It is said to be much more potent than other anti-HIV NRTI agents and seems active against phenotypically and/or genotypically NRTI-resistant HIV strains. Antiretroviral activity of stampidine in cats chronically infected with

FIV has also been studied. Notably, a single oral bolus dose of stampidine resulted in a significant decrease in the FIV load of circulating PBMCs in five of six FIV-infected cats [166]. Its antiretroviral properties in NRTI-resistant HIV strains, together with its favorable animal toxicity profile, pharmacokinetics, and *in vivo* antiretroviral activity in FIV-infected cats renders stampidine a promising new NRTI compound.

Similarly to the nucleoside analogs, the target enzyme of NNRTIs is also the viral RT. In contrast to the NRTIs, NNRTIs are not «false» building blocks, but rather attach directly and non-competitively to the enzyme, at a position in close proximity to the substrate binding site for nucleosides. The resulting complex can thus bind fewer nucleosides, slowing polymerization down significantly. In contrast to the nucleoside class of inhibitors, NNRTIs are highly specific for HIV-1, and they are not active against HIV-2 or any other retrovirus, including SIV and FIV. Indeed, despite the high similarity of the NNRTI target sequence between HIV-1 RT and FIV RT, no inhibitory effect of NNRTIs against FIV RT has ever been reported, even at drug concentrations that are significantly higher than those required to fully suppress HIV-1 RT activity [167]. With the objective to map the determinants of the lack of susceptibility of FIV RT to anti- HIV-1 NNRTIs, Auwerx and colleagues constructed a variety of chimeric FIV RTs, equipping this enzyme with the amino acids that have been proven to engender susceptibility of HIV-1 RT toward NNRTIs [168]. This study revealed that profound differences between FIV RT and HIV-1 RT in terms of structure and/or flexibility are responsible for the absence of interaction of FIV RT with NNRTIs. Thus, to date, researchers have not yet succeeded in either transforming FIV RT to acquire susceptibility to the inhibitory effects of the NNRTI, or elaborating a NNRTI which efficiently binds and inhibits FIV RT.

The retroviral PR cuts the viral *gag-pol* polyprotein into its functional subunits. Thus, inhibition of the protease, preventing appropriate splicing and maturation of essential structural proteins, leads to the release of virus particles that are unable to infect new cells. With knowledge of the molecular structure of the protease encoded by HIV, the first protease inhibitors were designed in the early nineties.

However, the emergence of resistant strains, in which the sequence of the viral PR is altered in a way that leads to the impairment of inhibition, has grown rapidly problematic. Again, despite high structural homology of both proteases, FIV PR demonstrates poor binding of inhibitors in clinical use against HIV-1 PR. Several studies have shown that FIV PR contains, at equivalent positions, amino acid residues that are identical to those found in drug-resistant forms of HIV-1 PR. The PR structure of FIV was then used as a model for the development of a series of PIs with broad efficacy. Thus, the most potent FIV PI, designated TL-3, was able to block nearly 100% of virus production in an acute infection against HIV, FIV, and SIV *ex vivo*. Furthermore, it was not toxic to cells, and there was no sign of resistance development by the different viruses even after 2 months of culture [169]. *In vivo* in the domestic cat, TL-3 treatment engendered modest lowering of viral loads and greater survival rates in treated symptomatic animals at 8 weeks post-infection with a highly pathogenic FIV-C isolate [170]. Moreover, early TL-3 treatment was shown to effectively counteract FIV effects on the central nervous system (CNS) of infected cats as well as eliminate FIV-induced changes in the CNS [171]. Although continued treatment is required to lower average viral loads and to maintain unimpaired CNS function, TL-3 seems to have a considerable therapeutic effect against FIV infection.

Inhibition of FIV entry into host cells provides an exciting new and emerging approach for the development of antiviral therapies. The identification of the peptide sequences responsible for gp120/receptor binding allows the creation of a class of pharmaceuticals called fusion inhibitors, whose mechanism of action is to competitively antagonize virus binding. In 1996, Lombardi and colleagues, screened 20- to 23-mer peptides covering the entire *env* gene of FIV and found especially potent *in vitro* antiviral activity associated with a peptide referred to as peptide 59, derived from a region located in the ectodomain of the TM protein. Unfortunately, peptide 59 did not appear promising as a therapeutic strategy for naturally occurring infections since it could only inhibit tissue culture-adapted FIV in fibroblastoid cells (CRFK), but not a primary isolate in feline lymphoid cells [172]. Because the activity of peptide 59 mapped to a short sequence containing three conserved tryptophan

(Trp) residues, further analyses were carried out with a peptide of eight amino acids, designated C8, comprising such a Trp motif. Peptide C8, although rather unstable due to its reduced size, exerted a powerful antiviral effect *in vitro* on all the FIV isolates tested, and this activity was dependent on an intact Trp motif [173]. Further studies have demonstrated that the C8 retroinverso analog (riC8) possesses similar inhibitory potential and a much increased stability, maintaining its concentration unchanged for at least 24 hours in cat serum *in vitro*. Most exciting are the results of a short-term monotherapy experiment in chronically FIV-infected cats showing that riC8 is well tolerated and also has substantial antiviral activity *in vivo* [174].

Relatively new treatment perspectives focus on modulation of the host immune system, exploring the potential of various immunostimulatory cytokines and antioxidants. Immunomodulatory agents are probably the most widely used medications in FIV-infected cats.

In addition to their immunomodulatory effect, both type I and type II IFN also exhibit a direct antiviral effect by inducing in non-infected cells a general antiviral state, that protects them against virus replication. Strong inhibitory activity of human as well as feline type I IFN against FIV replication has been reported in an experiment testing *in vitro* treatment of a feline T cell line and feline PBMCs with either recombinant human interferon alpha (rHuIFN-α) or its corresponding feline interferon, the recombinant feline interferon omega (rFeIFN-ω) [61]. As interferons are species-specific, feline and human interferons clearly differ in both antigenicity and antiviral efficacy in feline cells. Thus, rHuINF-α showed insignificant effects on peripheral blood lymphocyte subsets in FIV-infected cats, and was clearly ineffective in immunodeficient animals, which exhibited severe lymphocyte depletion. Although monotherapy was thus excluded, rHuINF-α seemed however to demonstrate some clinical benefits with no side effects when used in complement to antibiotic and symptomatic therapy [175]. In contrast, rFeIFN-ω demonstrated significant therapeutic effects and increase in survival rate of cats with clinical signs associated with FeLV infection and FeLV/FIV co-infection [176].

The results of several studies concerning effect of human type II IFN (HuIFN-γ) on HIV replication remain to date controversial. FIV replication seems not to be inhibited by recombinant feline IFN gamma (rFeIFN-γ) in feline PBMCs, and rather enhanced in the FetJ feline T cell line [61]. This finding may be explained by the mostly indirect effects of IFN-γ *in vivo*, modulated by CTL and NK cell responses to virus-infected cells.

An additional cytokine, the recombinant human granulocyte-macrophage colony stimulating factor (rHuGMCSF), was recently evaluated for its antiviral effects in the course of FIV disease. Similar to its use in humans, rHuGMCSF can be used to increase the production and functional activity of neutrophils in animals with infectious disease. However, these drugs are not veterinary-labeled products and the potential risks must be considered in relation to the therapeutic benefits for veterinary use. Overall, rHuGMCSF treatment increased neutrophil counts in FIV-infected cats without affecting the infection status. Furthermore, due to production of neutralizing antibodies to rHuGMCSF, and the possible development of cross-neutralizing antibodies to recombinant feline GMCSF, long term treatment with rHuGMCSF may induce severe adverse reactions and is not recommended in cats [177].

Another explored route was the therapeutic potential of several immunosuppressive drugs on FIV. Indeed, as immune activation may lead to increased FIV replication, an attractive treatment hypothesis has been to suppress the immune system in an attempt to interfere with viral replication and apoptosis of host cells. Although glycocorticoids were shown to enhance the course of infection [178], two potent immunosuppressive drugs, Cylosporine A and Tacrolimus, commonly utilized in preventing graft rejection following organ transplantation, have proved to protect cells against apoptosis and decrease virus production in both acutely and chronically infected cats [179]. Use of both immunosuppressants and immunostimulants in the therapeutic setting shows the clear discrepancy between defined and hypothetical scientific knowledge, and highlights the current difficulties encountered in further development of drugs suitable for treatment of FIV.

Literature

Despite numerous studies, clinical use of antiviral drugs is still not very common in veterinary medicine. Many antiviral drugs that have been experimentally tested never appear on the market due to high toxicity. With the exception of the new feline IFN-ω that is now on the market in some European countries and Japan, no antiviral drugs are licensed for veterinary medicine. Therefore, attempts to treat an FIV-infected cat must be carried out with human drugs such as AZT.

3.1.8 Prevention

3.1.8.1 General Considerations

Although ethically questioned in areas of low FIV prevalence, keeping cats indoors to avoid contact with homeless, feral, abandoned or stray cats is the most effective mode of prevention against infection. Outdoor cats should ideally be neutered, in order to diminish territorial behaviour and transmission during mating. Additionally, testing of new cats before introduction in a FIV-seronegative household is crucial. Infected cats should be housed indoors at all times to avoid infection of FIV-naive cats and to lessen their own risks to acquire opportunistic infections. Finally, although the transmission efficacy from queens to kittens is low during the asymptomatic phase of disease, kittens of FIV-infected queens should optimally not be allowed to nurse in order to avoid transmission by ingestion of milk.

3.1.8.2 Vaccination

Vaccine development is essential, in order to protect the pet cat population from FIV infection and to control the high worldwide prevalence within reservoir stray cat populations. Furthermore, promising FIV vaccine designs may serve as models for the identification of effective prophylactic treatments to HIV. The development of lentiviral vaccines remains however a real challenge, due to the viral affection of important host immune components. A healthy immune system is indeed crucial for efficient vaccine immunity. Cellular tropism of FIV for T and B cell populations as well as for the monocyte/macrophage system renders the development of an efficacious product extremely difficult.

In addition to their complex pathogenesis, lentiviruses are known for their mutative potential and their diversity in the field. The various FIV subtypes differ typically in antigenic properties recognized by the immune system, which are, as a consequence, also targeted by vaccine studies. The development of a vaccine which harbours potency against several, or ideally all subtypes of FIV, is crucial to clinical utility in the field, and remains an ongoing challenge.

Efficacious lentiviral vaccine development has indeed revealed itself particularly tricky. Many factors influence greatly the outcome of individual studies, and it is crucial to take them into consideration when criticizing the different attempts elaborated over time. Overall, technical differences in vaccine inactivation procedure and composition, such as cell types used for growing vaccine virus, vaccination schedule, adjuvant used, vaccine doses, and variable virulence between FIV strains have produced conflicting results over time. The analysis of some important influencing factors in vaccine studies is detailed below.

3.1.8.2.1 Choice of Adjuvant

An important facet of vaccine production is the selection of an appropriate adjuvant. Although these substances have no specific antigenic effect, their presence in the composition of a vaccine reduces the amount of antigen needed to achieve the desired immune response, increasing potency of immunization, and lowering cost in vaccine production.

In the search of a vaccine for infections with a complexe pathogenesis such as lentiviral infections, the conjunction of an adjuvant may obviously play a determinig role in the success of the immunization trial.

Different adjuvants are chemically highly heterogenous and affect the immune system in various ways. Their mode of action generally consists in formation of a gradually released depot of antigen at the site of inoculation, presentation of antigen and stimulation of immunocompetent cells, as well as production of various lymphokines and immunoglobulins. Due to the resultant hyperactivation of the host's immune system, they may however induce variably serious side effects. In cats, the occurence of vaccine-related fibrosarcoma, an especially malignant cancer originating from fibrous connective tissue at the site of vaccine injection, has grown to a serious concern in the past years. There is evidence that adjuvants play an inciting role in the formation of these deadly tumours. The choice of an adjuvant thus reflects a compromise between requirement for adjuvanticity and an acceptable level of adverse reactions.

Of all adjuvants tested in animal vaccine research, complete Freund's adjvant (CFA) probably remains the most well known. CFA is an aqueous antigen solution emulsified in mineral oil, composed of inactivated and dried mycobacteria, originally *Mycobacterium tuberculosis*, now mostly M.butyricum, stimulating cell-mediated immunity and leading to the potentiated production of certain immunoglobins. Due to its toxicity, its use in humans is forbidden, and there are currently a number of guidelines associated with its use in animal research. While usually effective, it may indeed induce undesirable side effects such as inflammation, induration, pain and necrosis at the injection site in mammals. These facts have led to refinement of its use and development of alternatives.

In FIV vaccine trials, a variety of alternatives to Freund's adjuvant have been tested. In this way, incomplete Freund's adjuvant (IFA), lacking killed mycobacteria which represent the most inflammatory component of CFA, was initially used for boosting immunizations subsequent to primary vaccination combined with CFA. It may also serve for initial immunization, particularly in combination with a « strong » antigen. Similarly, the minimal chemical structure from the mycobacterium in CFA, the peptidoglycan muramyl dipeptide (MDP), provides adjuvant activity and its use significantly decreases the disadvantages encountered with CFA. Moreover, when MDP was incorporated into incomplete Freund's adjuvant it was found to replace completely the adjuvant activity of the mycobacterium. MDP was also found to have adjuvant activity when used alone. Although its pyrogenic potential remains a limiting factor in its use as adjuvant, MDP has been used in various forms and combinations in FIV vaccine studies.

Oil-in-water emulsions represent another class of widely used adjuvants. The Ribi adjuvant, for example, contains detoxified endotoxin with mycobacterial cell wall components. It presents very low toxicity and is as convenient to use as Freund's complete adjuvant, due to its low viscosity. Similarly, Syntex Adjuvant Formulation (SAF) is a stabilized oil-in-water emulsion known to activate complement by the alternate pathway. SAF was used quite successfully in early vaccine studies when combined to various forms of MDP.

Mineral compounds are also of common use for supplementation of vaccine antigens. Aluminium hydroxide, for example, allows particularly slow release of the antigen at the injection site, prolonging the time for interaction between antigen and antigen presenting cells and lymphocytes. Its use in cats however has been very controversial, as this agent has been speculated to play an important role in the induction of lethal tumours at the injection site.

Plant-derived chemicals have also been tested in their adjuvanticity for FIV vaccines. Quil-A, a highly refined form of saponin, was also shown to stimulate both cell-mediated and humoral immune responses. Additionally, it serves as the main component of immune stimulating complexes called ISCOMs, relatively stable but non-covalently bound complexes of Quil-A, cholesterol and amphipathic antigen. The main characteristic of ISCOM-associated antigen molecules is that they are transported to the draining lymph nodes and thus do not deposit at site of injection. Furthermore, very low quantities of antigen can elicit a significant immune response, thus rendering the use of ISCOMs an interesting approach to stimulation of the host immune response towards amphipathic antigens. ISCOMs have only been used in veterinary vaccines, partly due to their haemolytic activity and some local reactions, all reflecting the detergent activity of the Quil-A molecule.

A new class of adjuvants has arised with the introduction of DNA vaccination, which enables co-delivery of specific antigens and molecular adjuvants, such as cytokines or unmethylated CpG ODN motifs, as an attempt to favourably alter

Literature

initial immune events in infection. Indeed, the earliest antiviral defences are innate, and provide the basis on which the subsequent adaptive immune response is built. Moreover, further study of lentiviral pathogenesis has enabled characterization of unfavourable alterations or insufficient host response, which take place soon after the onset of infection, indicating the importance of influencing the innate immunity in the development of effective lentiviral vaccines. In this way, co-expression of vaccine antigens with cytokines abnormally produced in the early events of infection, such as IL-12 and IL-16, have indicated promising results. Similarly, CpG motifs, comprised of unmethylated CG dinucleotides flanked by two 5' purines and two 3' pyrimidines, directly activate monocytes, macrophages, and dentritic cells to secrete IL-12 and IFN-γ. Their utility has been demonstrated for a variety of antigens, and they initiated convincing results as adjuvants in DNA vaccines [180]. Further characterization of CpG ODNs as well as their effects on the immune system are thouroughly described in the second chapter of this literature overview (3.2).

Unfortunately, no independent experiments comparing a wide variety of adjuvants with each other have been carried out so far. Only individual studies using certain adjuvant combinations allow limited comparison of the different existing adjuvant types and combinations. Thus, at the current stage of FIV vaccine development, there are no general conclusions as to which adjuvant formulation is more effective.

3.1.8.2.2 Importance of Challenge Methods

The evaluation of vaccine efficacy should readily take into consideration the challenge conditions. Indeed, the outcome of the study is greatly influenced by features such as quantity and virulence of the strain used, number of subtypes tested, source of the challenge inoculum and challenge route.

Since possibly no vaccine may be able to provide complete protection against a high-dose challenge or a highly virulent strain, these situations require modifications in the standards of judging vaccine efficacy. Generally, vaccines are designed to provide immunity capable of destroying all traces of virus in the host. Preclinical studies have however demonstrated that protection against disease is easier to achieve than prevention of infection. Critical evaluation of a vaccine study should be based on the observed effects on hallmarks of active infection, such as virus load, CD4+ counts, CD4+/CD8+ ratio, CD8+ cytotoxic activity, and specific FIV antibody titre, as well as the duration of positive alterations. Although the achievements of studies which failed to demonstrate sterilizing immunity are considered insufficient for clinical use, induction of partial immunity in presence of a severe challenge system nevertheless represents a great step towards the finding of an efficacious vaccine.

Many studies indicate efficient protection against infection with a homologous strain. However, due to the genetic variability of the different FIV subtypes, the demonstration of protection against both homologous and heterologous challenges has become a standard feature in FIV vaccine development. Multi-subtype vaccines not only broaden immunity and protection, but seem to have a synergistic protective potential. In this sense, several dual subtype vaccines have been tested for veterinary use against FIV infection. In 2002, the United States department of Agriculture approved Fel-O-Vax FIV, a dual subtype FIV vaccine, for commercial use. More details concerning the first vaccine against FIV ever released on the market are discussed in section 3.1.8.2.4.2.

Vaccine prophylaxis is also influenced by the source of the challenge inoculum. Studies suggest that homologous FIV vaccines using *in vitro*-produced antigen may not provide protection against challenges using *in vivo*-derived inoculum [181]. *In vitro* challenge material is a laboratory grown primary PBMC inoculum, cell free and purified, which can be readily produced at high titres, in large quantities, and at a relatively low cost. This method is thus commonly used for the screening of potential vaccines. *In vivo*-derived inoculum consists of plasma or infected cells derived from cats infected with *in vivo*-passaged laboratory isolates, which contain quasi-species of FIV and more closely simulate natural conditions. This approach, however, encounters multiple limitations in inoculum production and achievement of high titres, and is associated with increased costs. Furthermore, biological effects of the plasma or the cellular component of the inoculum are more variable among the recipient animals, in comparison to *in vitro*-derived inoculum.

At last, it is important to take the route of challenge into consideration when judging results of a vaccine study. Conventional methods include subcutaneous (s.c), intramuscular (i.m), intraperitoneal (i.p), intravenous (i.v) and mucosal exposures. It is still controversial which route most closely mimics the natural infection route of biting and fighting. However, it is known that i.v and i.p routes readily infect cats, whereas the s.c and mucosal routes require higher challenge doses. Since the level of the FIV exposure during natural transmission remains unknown, the efficacy evaluation using a contact challenge system represents the ultimate test for any commercial FIV vaccine. According to contact studies and epidemiological surveys, contact transmission of FIV requires long term exposure (months to years) to naturally infected cats, and disease manifestation is not common during the early phases of natural infection. These observations support the hypothesis that natural transmission occurs at low doses [182]. Although this method most closely mimics natural conditions, it remains extremely complicated to carry out experimentally in a representative form. As natural strains differ from the more thoroughly studied laboratory strains, questions arise concerning the dose requirements for occurrence of natural transmission, the virulence of the strains present in naturally infected populations, and their potential to maintain high viral loads in body fluids over time. In addition to obvious time and cost issues, these obstacles question the feasibility of natural transmission studies for commercial vaccine validation. However, in order to improve the quality of newly produced promising vaccines, the recourse to such studies will become difficult to circumvent.

3.1.8.2.3 Immune Correlates of Protection and Passive Immunity

Passive transfer of protection plays a less important role in FIV than in HIV disease, where preventing infection after accidental exposure to the virus or interrupting transmission of virus from mother to child demands efficacious post-exposure prophylaxy possibilities. Although clinical use of passive immunization remains insignificant in the case of FIV, several studies concerning passive immunity have allowed the characterization of important mechanisms in FIV vaccine protection.

Hohdatsu and co-workers evaluated the role of antiviral antibodies by passive immunization against experimental infection [183]. In this study, cats immunized with sera from either FIV-infected or FIV-vaccinated cats were protected from infection. Furthermore, maternal antiviral antibodies, including VN antibodies, from either infected or vaccinated queens were shown to protect neonatal kittens from FIV inoculation. Thus, maternal antiviral antibodies play a key role in preventing or limiting infection in neonates and vaccinated queens can provide such antiviral immunity [184].

In another study, cats were either passively immunized with serum-derived antibodies or transfused with peripheral blood cells from FIV-vaccinated cats. In both cases, the immunized animals were protected against an FIV challenge which infected all control cats, suggesting that not only humoral, but also cell-mediated immunity from vaccinated animals can protect naive animals upon experimental FIV challenge [185]. The role of cellular immunity in vaccine protection against FIV infection was further evaluated using adoptive cell transfer studies. It could be demonstrated, that protection mediated by adoptive transfer of immunocytes from vaccinated cats was MHC-restricted, occurred in the absence of antiviral humoral immunity, and correlated with the transfer of cells with FIV-specific CTL and T helper activities [186]. Thus, both humoral and cellular immunity seem to be able to individually confer protection against homologous challenge and should be, as a consequence, induced together for optimal vaccine protection.

3.1.8.2.4 FIV Vaccine Trials

3.1.8.2.4.1 Generalities

Whole virus vaccines, live or killed, constitute the vast majority of vaccines in use at present, in both human and veterinary medicine. Approaches using attenuated live retroviral vaccines are considered to be impractical for clinical trials in humans, due to risk of reversion to virulence. In FIV vaccine trials however, the highest levels of success has been achieved with inactivated whole virus or inactivated infected-cell vaccines. Heat, chemical or irradiation methods thereby render the virus completely non-infectious. It is important to note that since they are incapable of replicating in the host, inactivated vaccines require larger amounts of antigen, and require multiple doses as well as the use of an appropriate adjuvant for optimal efficacy.

Recent advances in molecular biology have provided alternative methods for producing vaccines. The technology enabling growth of viruses to high titres in cell cultures has enabled purification of virus and viral antigens. Furthermore, the identification of important peptides encompassing the major antigenic sites of important viral proteins allows the production of highly purified subunit vaccines. Specific viral proteins can be expressed in bacteria, yeast, mammalian cells, and other viruses, and used as recombinant vectored vaccines. An additional interesting development has been the production of synthetic peptides closely mimicking specific viral immunogenic sites. The antigens of synthetic peptide vaccines are precisely defined and free from unnecessary components which may be associated with side effects. Overall, the production and quality control of such subunit vaccines is simple, and this technique is considered safe with viruses which establish a persistent infection. Increasing purification may lead to loss of immunogenicity however, and this often induces the necessity of coupling the purified peptides to an immunogenic carrier protein. Furthermore, the induced immunogenic response is restricted to selected antigens and vaccination of this type may not provide significant protection against natural challenge.

DNA vaccines represent another recently developed method in use for vaccine trials. They usually comprise circular plasmids that include a gene encoding the target antigens. This gene is under the transcriptional control of a promoter region active in specific host cells, which then directly produce the foreign antigen. DNA vaccines offer greater control over the immunization process, because the investigator determines which antigens and co-stimulants to use, where to elicit the response, and whether to use immunostimulatory DNA sequences to modulate the type of immune response induced. In addition, DNA is relatively inexpensive and easier to produce than conventional vaccines. Safety issues with regard to DNA vaccines include risks of integration into cellular DNA and antibiotic resistance conferred through resistance genes present in the plasmid. However, only insignificant adverse reactions have been noted so far in the many preclinical trials carried out with such vaccines, and this method remains very promising for future studies.

The following chapters describe different strategic approaches to protection against lentiviral infection, as well as encountered difficulties, in a series of relevant FIV vaccine studies performed mainly in the last 10 years. Tables 5-7 give detailed information about the individual studies.

3.1.8.2.4.2 Conventional Vaccines

The main concern in the use of inactivated whole virus or inactivated infected cell vaccines is the event of accidental infection caused by incomplete inactivation of the vaccine virus. Thus, alternative methods were more thoroughly investigated for the development of prophylactic measures against HIV. However, results from animal studies with inactivated vaccines can provide new insights into the immune mechanisms of protection against lentiviruses. Such conventional vaccines have indeed achieved the majority of success in experimental FIV vaccine trials against severe challenge systems.

Several studies aimed at determining breadth of protection following immunization with a single strain inactivated whole virus vaccine. The first successful vaccine trial, reported in 1991, described efficient protection of a whole inactivated vaccine derived from FIV-PET, against an *in vitro*-derived homologous strain [187]. Further developing this study, Hosie et al. tested whether vaccination of cats with

FIV-PET could induce protection against homologous (FIV-PET) or heterologous (FIV-GL8) challenge [188]. Although both challenge virus strains belong to the FIV clade A, they present significant antigenic differences. As a consequence, vaccinated cats became infected following FIV-GL8 challenge. Later on however, the same group showed that inactivated FIV-PET vaccination significantly suppressed viral load and CD4+ T cell loss in cats challenged with FIV-GL8 [189]. In contrast, inactivated FIV-M2, a clade B FIV, conferred protection only following mucosal, and not systemic challenge using a primary homologous virus isolate [190]. Similarly, Pu et al. could not demonstrate efficient protection of cats vaccinated with whole inactivated clade D FIV (FIV-SHI) against homologous *in vivo*-derived challenge [181]. These results suggest that protection against an *in vivo*-derived homologous strain inoculum is difficult to achieve with single-strain immunizations.

Single-subtype infected fixed cell vaccines seem to confer protection at best against homologous challenge strains. Various cell types have been experimented over the years for their immunogenic potential as part of a vaccine. Infected cell vaccines derived from thymocyte or CRFK fibroblasts were not effective even against low dose, *in vitro*-derived homologous challenges [191]. Overall, successful cell-derived conventional vaccines have been developed from infected feline T lymphocyte cell lines. Greater than 90% protection was observed with a vaccine derived from chronically FIV-PET (subtype A) infected FL-4, an IL-2 independent feline T cell line, against *in vitro*-derived homologous and slightly heterologous challenge inoculums [192]. In a similar study, Matteucci and colleagues demonstrated homologous protection of cats after vaccination with FIV-M2 (subtype B) infected MBM cells, an IL-2 dependent feline T lymphoblastoid cell line developed by the same group in 1995 [193]. A study experimenting immunization with autologous FIV-M2 infected lymphoblasts however failed to show efficient protection, even against a low dose of homologous *ex vivo* FIV challenge [194].

The lack of heterologous protection of single subtype inactivated infected-cell or whole vaccines led to the multi-subtype vaccine approach, aiming at broadening immunity and protection. The first dual subtype FIV vaccine, consisting of inactivated subtype A- and D-infected cells, provided protection against *in vitro* derived homologous strains, but was unfortunately not tested against heterologous strains [195]. An improved dual-subtype FIV vaccine, consisting of inactivated whole viruses of subtypes A and D, elicited strong anti-FIV cellular immunity and broad spectrum VN antibody activities. In addition, it provided protection of cats against homologous and heterologous challenges using *in vivo*-derived inoculum [181]. This vaccine turned out to be the prototype of Fel-O-Vax FIV, a dual subtype vaccine produced with FIV subtypes A and D, and formulated with a proprietary adjuvant system, approved by the United States Department of Agriculture, and commercially released by Fort Dodge Animal Health in 2002. The efficacy of this vaccine was demonstrated in a vaccination study designed to meet various requirements for registering the vaccine [196]. Eight week old kittens were immunized with the vaccine, challenged 12 months later with a heterologous FIV strain, and monitored for FIV viremia. While 90% of the controls became persistently infected with FIV, only 16% of the vaccinated cats developed viremia, which demonstrated not only efficacy of the vaccine but also immunity against infection lasting for at least 12 months. The same study included a field safety trial in which 689 cats of various breeds, ages, and vaccination histories received a total of 2051 doses of the vaccine. Based on the fact that only 1% of the vaccinated cats presented mild reactions of short duration, the vaccine was considered safe for use in the field. Moreover, similarly to its prototype, which had demonstrated the potential to protect cats against heterologous challenge, Fel-O-Vax was shown to effectively protect cats against virulent challenge with a subtype B isolate, reported to be most common in the USA [197]. A contact study, more closely reflecting field conditions, confirmed these findings: 6 vaccinated and 8 control cats housed with 5 cats infected with a subtype B FIV strain were monitored for infection over several years. All vaccinated animals remained protected whereas 50% of the unvaccinated cats became infected, suggesting the vaccine exhibits broad efficacy against genetically diverse FIV strains, even under contact challenge [198]. Unfortunately, Fel-O-Vax has a major conflict with current FIV diagnostics, including ELISA and Western

Literature

Type of Immunization	Virus (FIV Subtype)	Vaccine Administration route	Protocol (weeks)	Type of Adjuvant
Whole Virus Pelleted	PET (A)	s.c.	0,2,4,7,10,17	T-MDP/SAF-M
	PET (A)	s.c.	0,2,4,7,10,17	T-MDP/SAF-M
Gradient purified Whole Virus	PET (A)	s.c.	0,3,6	T-MDP/SAF-M
	PET (A)	s.c.	0,3,6	T-MDP/SAF-M
Infected CrFK Cells	UT113 (A)	i.m.	0,3,6	G-MDP/H20/mineral oil
Infected Thymocytes	UT113 (A)	i.m.	0,3,6	G-MDP/H20/mineral oil
Infected MBM Cells	M-2 (B)	s.c.	0,3,6,9,21	IFA
Infected FL-4 Cells	Pet (A)	s.c.	0,4,8	A-MDP
	Pet (A) and SHI (D)	s.c.	0,4,8	A-MDP
Biotinylated Whole Virus	M-2 (B)	i.p.	0,4,8,12	Homol-RBC
	M-2 (B)	i.p.	0,4,8,12	Homol-RBC
	M-2 (B)	i.p.	0,4,8,12,16	Homol-RBC
	M-2 (B)	i.p.	0,4,8,12,16	Homol-RBC
Purified Whole Virus	M-2 (B)	s.c.	0,3,6,9,20	IFA
	M-2 (B)	s.c. (+ i.vag.)	0,3,6,9,20	IFA +/- CT
Purified Whole Virus	PET (A)	s.c.	0,3,6	MF59.0
	PET (A)	s.c.	0,3,6	MF59.0
	PET (A)	s.c.	0,3,6	MF59.0
Infected Fixed MBM Cells	M-2 (B)	s.c.	0,3,6,16,40,64	IFA
Whole Virus	Pet (A) and SHI (D)	s.c.	0,3,9	FD-1
	Pet (A) and SHI (D)	s.c.	0,3,9,12	FD-1
	Pet (A)	s.c.	0,3,9,12	FD-1
	SHI (D)	s.c.	0,3,9,12	FD-1

Table 5: Whole virus and infected-cell vaccine trials against FIV infection.

Challenge Inoculum		Protection Rate (No.inf/no.challenged)	Reference
Dose (CID50) and Strain (FIV Subtype)	Route of Administration		
10 PET (A)	i.p.	5/6	
5 GL-8 (A)	i.p.	0/5	188
10 PET (A)	i.p.	5/5	
5 GL-8 (A)	i.p.	1/5	
10 UT113 (A)	s.c.	0/5	191
10 UT113 (A)	s.c.	1/3	
10 M-2 (B)	i.v.	5/6	199
10 Pet (A) or Shi (D)	i.p.	0/4 and 3/4	195
10 Pet (A) or Shi (D)	i.p.	0/4 and 0/4	
10 M-2 (B)	i.v	4/4	
10 M-2 (B)	i.v	0/4	200
10 M-2 (B)	i.v.	0/4	
10 M-2 (B)	i.v.	0/4	
10 M-2 (B)	i.v.	11/16	190
M-2, 2X 10e4 cells	i.vag.	4/12	
10 PET (A)	i.p.	5/5	
10 GL-8 (A)	i.p.	2/5	189
10 AM-6 (A)	i.p.	3/5	
Field isolate	contact exposure	12/12	201
10 Bang (B)	i.v.	4/5	
10 PET (A)	i.v.	4/4	181
10 PET (A)	i.v.	1/5	
10 SHI (D)	i.v.	1/3	

Blot technologies. Indeed, this conventional inactivated FIV vaccine induces broad spectrum antibody production to different FIV proteins, with long lasting titers. This renders differentiation of infected and vaccinated cats possible only with more expensive methods such as PCR. As a consequence, an efficient test allowing detection of vaccination-specific antibodies still needs to be elaborated.

The precedent for using a whole virus vaccine in cats has been established with FeLV vaccination. No known cases of accidental infection due to improper inactivation of the virus have been reported with FeLV vaccines. With improved inactivation methods of vaccine virus and better adjuvant formulations, inactivated or killed vaccine approaches continue to be promising for future veterinary vaccine development.

3.1.8.2.4.3 Subunit Vaccines

Recombinant subunit vaccine trials include purified viral proteins, synthetic peptide and live viral or bacterial vector-based vaccines. Unfortunately, although such constructs induce high rates of cellular responses accompanied by antibodies aimed at specific targeted proteins, limited success has been obtained with this type of immunization against lentiviruses.

Many studies have based their trials on envelope antigens, as these are considered major targets of the immune system, and, as a consequence, represent appropriate vaccine components. The relative ease in production of satisfyingly pure products additionally renders recombinant envelope components especially attractive in use as immunogens for such studies. Furthermore, presence of antibodies specific for viral proteins that are not present in the vaccine allows clear discrepancy of seroconversion induced by natural infection from vaccine-induced humoral response. Thus, failure to induce protection against homologous and heterologous challenge infection despite induction of a considerable humoral response by highly purified denatured or native recombinant SU proteins originally expressed in the Baculovirus system and in E. coli, was both surprising and disappointing [202]. In an effort to increase the immune response and thus the protection rate observed in this study, recombinant SU proteins were further tested in a series of immunization trials assessing feasibility of combining these peptides with either QS-21 adjuvant or Freund's adjuvant together with the recombinant nucleocapsid protein of the rabies virus. Better results in this experiment indicated that conjunction of recombinant FIV SU with appropriate adjuvants leads to partial protection against FIV challenge infection [203]. With similar objectives, Hosie and co-workers tested immunoaffinity purified gp120 for its prophylactic potential in FIV infection [204]. Again, although immunized cats presented a lower viral load in PBMCs than control cats, this vaccine failed to confer complete protection following challenge. A more recent study, aiming at the determination of the level of crossreactivity between HIV-1 and FIV, demonstrated an overall protection rate of 78% against challenge FIV infection using *in vivo*-derived inocula of both subtype B and recombinant subtype A/B, in cats immunized with adjuvanted recombinant HIV-1 p24 [205]. A vaccine consisting of only HIV-1 protein thus appears to be efficacious against FIV infection, suggesting that the epitopes shared by members of the lentivirus family may have protective properties. Interestingly, such protection did not correlate with antibody titres, and Th1-promoting cytokines, supplemented in the adjuvant, greatly enhanced the HIV-1 p24 vaccine efficacy. These findings indicate that cross-protection observed in HIV-1 p24 vaccinated cats was most likely mediated by the cellular immunity. Future studies should determine whether the FIV-infected cat is a useful small animal AIDS model to characterize protective epitopes for HIV-1 vaccine design.

Another approach to development of subunit vaccines was the production of synthetic peptides. Again, most studies have based their immunization trials on envelope antigens, with limited success. Thus, immunization with a synthetic peptide, containing the immunodominant neutralization epitope located within the V3 domain of the FIV envelope glycoprotein, failed to confer protection in all of the immunized cats, although the peptide had induced both specific cell-mediated and

Literature

Type of Immunization	Virus (FIV Subtype)	Vaccine		Type of Adjuvant
		Administration route	Protocol (weeks)	
gp 100 (highly purified)	ZH-2 (A)	i.m.	0,2,4,8	AlOH/QS21
gp 100 (native)	ZH-2 (A)	i.m.	0,2,4,8	AlOH/QS21
gp 100 (highly purified)	Bang (B)	i.m.	0,2,4,8	AlOH/QS21
gp 100 (glycosylated)	Bang (B)	i.m.	0,2,4,8	AlOH/QS21
V3-Region Peptide	GL-8 (A)	s.c.	0,3,6	Quil A
Vectored- env	WO (A)	?	0,4,30	ISA 206
	WO (A)	?	0,4,30	ISA 708
env (cleavage site)	AM-19 (A)	s.c.	0,4,6,8,10	ISCOM
env (no cleavage site)	AM-19 (A)	s.c.	0,4,6,8,10	ISCOM
	AM-19 (A)	s.c.	0,4,10	Quil A
V3-Fusion Protein I	UT-113 (A)	s.c.	0,4,10	AlOH/oil
	UT-113 (A)	s.c.	0,4,10	AlOH/oil
Feline Herpes- env (+ boost V3-Peptide)	UT-113 (A)	oronasal/s.c. (boost i.m.)	0 (boost 4,8)	none (boost AlOH/oil)
	UT-113 (A)	oronasal/s.c. (boost i.m.)	0 (boost 4,8)	none (boost Quil A)
gp 120 (highly purified)	Pet (A)	s.c.	0,3,6,12	t-MDP/SAF-M
synthetic multiepitopic env, , SU/TM, p24, gag	Pet (A)	s.c.	0,3,6,15,19	Quil A
E.coli expressed SU	ZH-2 (A)	s.c.	0,2,4	AlOH + QS-21
Baculovirus expressed SU	ZH-2 (A)	s.c.	0,2,4	AlOH + QS-21
	ZH-2 (A)	s.c.	0,2,4	Freund's/AlOH/rabies N
VEE vector expressing env and gag	NCSU	s.c.	0,4,8,12,16,20	–
HIV p24	HIV-1 (UCD1)	s.c.	?	Ribi/rfeIL-12
HIV p24	HIV-1 (UCD1)	s.c.	?	Ribi/rfeIL-18
HIV p24	HIV-1 (UCD1)	?	?	Ribi/rfeIL-12

Table 6: Subunit vaccine trials against FIV infection.

Literature

Challenge Inoculum Dose (CID50) and Strain (FIV Subtype)	Route of Administration	Protection Rate (No.inf/no.challenged)	Reference
20 ZH-2 (A)	i.p.	0/5	201
20 ZH-2 (A)	i.p.	1/5	
20 ZH-2 (A)	i.p.	1/5	
20 ZH-2 (A)	i.p.	0/5	
20 PET (A)	i.p.	0/3	205
20 WO (A)	i.p.	0/4	207
20 WO (A)	i.p.	0/4	
20 AM-19 (A)	i.m.	0/6	211
20 AM-19 (A)	i.m.	0/6	
20 AM-19 (A)	i.m.	0/6	
0-20 UT-113 (A)	s.c.	0/5	208
0-20 UT-113 (A)	s.c.	0/5	
0-20 UT-113 (A)	s.c.	0/5	
0-20 UT-113 (A)	s.c.	0/5	
10 PET (A)	s.c.	1/5	203
25 PET (A)	i.p.	0/5	206
20 ZH-2 (A)	i.p.	0/5	202
20 ZH-2 (A)	i.p.	0/5	
20 ZH-2 (A)	i.p.	0/5	
5x10e5 NCSU-inf. PBMC and CD4E cells	i.vag.	0/8	209
15 BANG (A)	i.v.	4/4	204
15 BANG (A)	i.v.	2/3	
15 FCV1 (B)	i.v.	3/4	

humoral immune responses [206]. In the same way, cats immunized with a 46-residue multiepitopic synthetic peptide of FIV, comprising immunodominant epitopes present in V3 of the envelope glycoprotein, TM glycoprotein, and p24 *gag* core protein, developed an elaborate humoral immune response, but were not protected against challenge infection [207]. Synthetic peptides seem to be more effective *in vitro* however, as Lombardi and colleagues demonstrated a remarkable specific antiviral effect against the homologous and heterologous isolates using antibodies induced by synthetic peptides representing either a conserved region of the SU protein, or a hypervariable region of the TM protein [172].

Live recombinant vector vaccines are able to present the desired viral proteins in native conformation more efficiently than the purified subunit vaccines, and thereby elicit an immunity that may be more effective. The choice of a vector system that optimally expresses the desired proteins remains however challenging. Similar to the purified and synthesized subunit vaccines, envelope amino acids remain the protective epitopes of choice. A recombinant replication-defective vaccine composed of adenovirus type 5 vector expressing FIV *env* gene, was found to be ineffective at inducing *env*-specific antibody responses and at protecting cats against homologous infection [208]. Disappointing results were also reported using a FIV mutant expressing the FIV *env* gene. Despite several booster immunizations, FIV-specific antibody responses in vaccinated cats were only weak, and the vaccinates did not withstand challenge with a low dose of homologous virus [209]. Recently, Burkhard and colleagues used Venezuelan equine encephalitis (VEE) virus replicon particles to generate FIV *gag* and *env* expressing vaccine vectors [210]. Despite induction of innate as well as FIV-specific immune responses, all cats became infected following vaginal challenge with high dose, pathogenic cell-associated FIV-NCSU. Immunized cats, however, indicated a significantly lower drop of CD4+ cell counts after FIV infection. The best results in vaccination against FIV with a vector-based system came from a recombinant canarypoxvirus (ALVAC) based vaccine [211]. In this study, 2 of 3 cats immunized with the ALVAC FIV recombinants were protected from homologous FIV challenge in the presence of FIV-specific

CTL responses, but in the absence of FIV-specific humoral responses. Moreover, all 3 cats immunized with the ALVAC FIV recombinant and boosted with FIV- infected cell vaccine were protected from homologous FIV challenge in the presence of both FIV-specific CTL and humoral responses. This vaccine combination also induced partial protection against a heterologous challenge, which took place 8 months after the initial challenge. In conclusion, ALVAC indicates more promising results than other vector systems for FIV vaccine studies, and immunization schemes employing ALVAC vector in combination with inactivated FIV-infected cell vaccine can generate protective immune responses capable of crossreacting with FIV isolates that are genetically distinct from the vaccine strains.

3.1.8.2.4.4 DNA Vaccines

In the 1990s, DNA-mediated immunization emerged as a promising alternative in the development of viral vaccines, displaying protective immunity against viral and non-viral pathogens. This method had mainly attracted interest in lentiviral research for its potential to elicit strong cellular activity. Various trials effectively succeeded in reduction of viral load and prevention of disease after challenge, however complete protection was not achieved in either the HIV- or SIV-infected non-human primate models or FIV-infected domestic cats.

The most common approach to DNA vaccination trials has been the generation of live attenuated viruses with replication defective but full length proviral genomes, which express both structural and regulatory proteins *in vivo*. Moreover, inclusion of cytokine genes into a DNA vaccine enables increase of its immunogenicity and allows induction of desired types of immune responses. In 1998, Hosie and colleagues were the first to test DNA vaccination in the FIV model [213]. They vaccinated cats with a FIV mutant containing an in-frame deletion in *pol* (FIVΔRT), adjuvanted or not with INF-γ DNA. Altogether, the immunization with FIVΔRT elicited cytotoxic T cell responses to FIV *gag* and *env* in the absence of a serological response. After challenge with homologous virus, 4 of the 10 vaccinates remained

Literature

Type of Immunization	Virus (FIV Subtype)	Vaccine Administration route	Protocol (weeks)	Type of Adjuvant
Proviral FIVdRT	PET (A)	i.m.	0,10,23	-
	PET (A)	i.m.	0,10,23	feline IFNg DNA
Proviral FIVdRT	PET (A)	i.m.	0,4,8	feline IFNg DNA
	GL-8 (A)	i.m.	0,4,8	feline IFNg DNA
	PET (A)	i.m.	0,4,8	feline IFNg DNA
	GL-8 (A)	i.m.	0,4,8	feline IFNg DNA
Proviral FIVdVif	PPR (A)	i.m.	0,43	-
gp 140 DNA MIDGE	ZH-2	i.e.	0,3,6	feline IL-12 DNA MIDGE
	ZH-2	i.e.	0,3,6	feline IL-12 DNA MIDGE
	ZH-2	i.e.	0,3,6	CpGs
Proviral FIVdIN	GL-8 (A)	i.m.	0,4,8	-
	GL-8 (A)	i.m.	0,4,8	feline IL-18 DNA
	GL-8 (A)	i.m.	0,4,8	feline IL-12/IL-18 DNA
Proviral FIVdRT	GL-8 (A)	i.m.	0,4,8	feline IL-18 DNA
	GL-8 (A)	i.m.	0,4,8	feline IL-12/IL-18 DNA
Proviral FIVdIN	GL-8 (A)	i.m.	0,4,8,32	feline IL-18 DNA
	GL-8 (A)	i.m.	0,4,8,32	feline IL-12/IL-18 DNA
	GL-8 (A)	i.m.	0,4,8,32	feline IL-18 DNA
Proviral FIVdRT	GL-8 (A)	i.m.	0,4,8,32	feline IL-12/IL-18 DNA
Proviral FIVdIN	GL-8 (A)	i.m.	0,32	-
	GL-8 (A)	i.m.	0,32	feline IL-18 DNA
	GL-8 (A)	i.m.	0,32	feline IL-12/IL-18 DNA
Proviral FIVdOrf-A	Pet (A)	s.c.	28 weeks prior to challenge	-

Table 7: DNA vaccine trials against FIV infection.

Challenge Inoculum		Protection Rate	Reference
Dose (CID50) and Strain (FIV Subtype)	Route of Administration	(No.inf/no.challenged)	
25 PET (A)	?	1/5	212
25 PET (A)	?	3/5	
10 PET (A)	?	1/6	189
10 PET (A)	?	2/6	
10 GL-8 (A)	?	0/6	
10 GL-8 (A)	?	0/6	
PPR (A)	i.p.	5/5	6
25 TCID50 ZH-2 (A)	i.p.	3/4	215, 180
25 TCID50 ZH-2 (A)	i.p.	0/4	
25 TCID50 ZH-2 (A)	i.p.	0/4	
25 PET (A)	i.p.	1/6	213 (Study 1)
25 PET (A)	i.p.	2/6	
25 PET (A)	i.p.	2/6	
25 PET (A)	i.p.	2/6	
25 PET (A)	i.p.	0/6	
25 PET (A)	i.p.	1/1	213 (Study 2)
25 PET (A)	i.p.	2/2	
25 PET (A)	i.p.	1/1	
25 PET (A)	i.p.	0/1	
25 PET (A)	i.p.	0/1	213 (Study 3)
25 PET (A)	i.p.	0/2	
25 PET (A)	i.p.	0/1	
10 PET (A)	i.v.	3/9	214

seronegative and virus free, while the rest displayed significantly lower proviral and viral loads. Conjunction of INF-γ DNA in the vaccine increased the protection rate. Unfortunately, further studies failed to demonstrate protection potential of this FIV mutant against heterologous strains and more virulent challenges, thus excluding its possible utility in the field [189]. In the same way, FIV mutants containing an in-frame deletion in the integrase gene (FIVΔIN) conferred protection against homologous, but not heterologous challenge [214].

A FIV mutant containing deletions in the viral accessory gene *vif* (FIVΔvif) [6] or in the *orf-A* gene (FIVΔorf-A) [215], also indicated significant protection against homologous challenge. Again, these mutants induced mostly specific cellular responses in the host, although anti-*env* and anti-*gag* antibodies were isolated in several cats. In both studies, no reversion to wild type virus occurred in the vaccinated cats, indicating relative safety in this type of viral attenuation for use as vaccine. Unfortunately, efficacy against genetically diverse strains was not tested, thus not allowing definitive conclusions about their relevance in the field.

As attempt to increase efficiency in expression of the incorporated genes, other vaccine trials have experimented the gene gun bombardment as vaccine DNA delivery. Such inoculations occur intradermally, whereby DNA-coated gold beads are directly shot into the keratinocyte nucleus. Advantages of this method include requirement of only low amounts of DNA and constant efficiency of transfection, with relative independence of vaccine dose from the size of the animal. In 2000, Boretti and colleagues immunized cats by the ballistic transfer of gold particles coated with minimalistic, immunogenic defined gene expression (MIDGE) vectors coding for FIV surface and partial transmembrane proteins, complemented or not with feline IL-12 DNA. These vectors consisted of the double-stranded expression sequence flanked by a phosphorylated oligodeoxynucleotide hairpin sequence on both ends. MIDGE particles thus lack sequence elements present on conventional plasmid constructs that could compromise the safety and immunological efficacy of the vaccine. Interestingly, 3 out of 4 cats immunized with MIDGE containing FIV *env*-coding particles together with IL-12 DNA were protected against homologous challenge. Indeed, only one cat in this group became provirus positive, displaying however a greatly reduced viral load [216]. These findings suggest that FIV DNA vaccines, in combination with feline IL-12 DNA, may provide a promising way of inducing a protective immune response against FIV infection.

3.1.8.2.5 Enhancement Problem

Viruses initiate infection by attaching to host cells via interaction between viral surface proteins and specific receptor/co-receptor molecules on target cells. Antibodies specific for the viral surface proteins often inhibit this step of the infection cycle, resulting in reduced infectivity, and inducing so-called virus neutralization. In some circumstances, such antibodies have been shown to potentiate viral infection. This phenomenon is known as antibody-dependant enhancement (ADE). Different mechanisms of ADE have been thoroughly described for several virus-cell systems *in vitro*; however *in vivo* relevance of ADE remains unclear. Obviously, further characterization of ADE is of great interest in the understanding of the pathogenesis of diverse viral diseases.

Several studies have focused on the importance of ADE in retroviral infections. At least three different mechanisms (figure 6) for ADE of HIV infection *in vitro* have been hypothesized: a) interaction between antibody and cellular Fc receptor (FcR), b) interaction between the cellular complement receptor (CR) and the complement factors, induced by activation of the classical complement pathway during viral infection, and c) antibody or soluble factor induced conformational change in viral envelope, leading to activation of the glycoprotein and facilitating membrane fusion. Interestingly, it seems viral infection through ADE uses a more efficient intracellular viral replication pathway, which suppresses expression of antiviral genes such as tumour necrosis factor and inducible nitric oxide synthase (figure 6). Unfortunately, clinical significance of all types of ADE in HIV infection remains very controversial.

Literature

In the case of FIV, both antibody dependent and independent responses have been associated with viral replication enhancement, thus complicating the understanding of immune processes and the development of vaccines. In 1992, Hosie and co-workers vaccinated cats either with purified FIV incorporated into ISCOMs, recombinant FIV p24 ISCOMs, or a fixed, inactivated cell vaccine in Quil A adjuvant, and thereby observed a more rapid viremia in vaccinated cats compared to control cats [217]. Group-related elevated or low titers of anti-p24, anti-*env* and neutralizing antibodies in the vaccinated cats seemed to play no role in the outcome of the challenge. Instead, 100% of the vaccinated cats became viraemic compared with 78% of the controls. In the same way, vaccination with fixed autologous FIV-infected cells did not protect cats against challenge infection despite induction of FIV-specific humoral responses. Again, accelerated virus replication was observed [218].

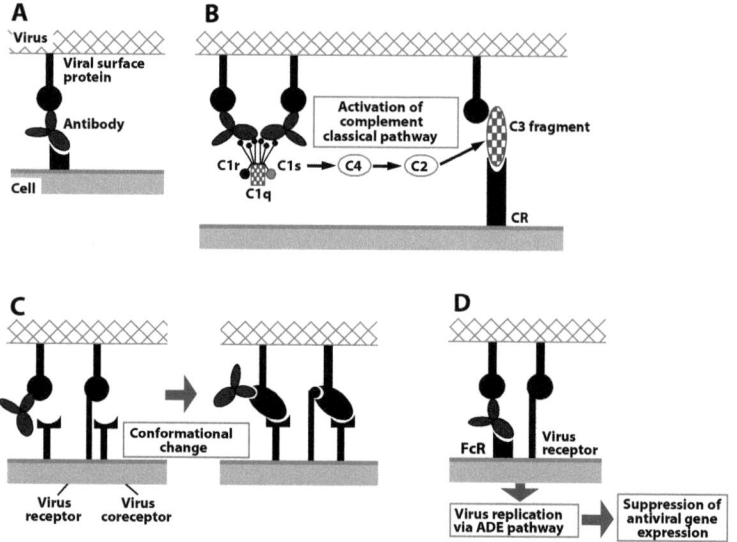

Figure 6: Mechanisms of antibody-dependent enhancement (see text for explanations)

When analyzing such results, it is important to keep in mind that whether antibodies enhance or neutralize seems to depend on the balance between various factors, including virus strain and dose, host-cell antibody combination, and the concentration and epitope-specificity of the antibody.

Further studies have focused on the importance of the retroviral envelope in enhancement, as it is known to be the principal target for viral neutralizing antibodies. Indeed, the majority of promising HIV vaccines undergoing clinical trials have been based on the viral envelope. However, monoclonal antibodies directed against a conserved region of the HIV TM glycoprotein, called the principal immunodominant domain (PID), were shown to induce enhancement of infection on several cell types, thus raising concern about the efficacy of such vaccines. In this sense, immunization of cats with recombinant vaccinia virus-expressed FIV envelope glycoprotein, either incorporated in ISCOMS or adjuvanted with Quil A, resulted in enhanced infectivity of FIV. Additionally, as the observed enhancement could be transferred to naive cats with plasma collected at the day of challenge, the authors proposed that enhancement was mediated by anti-*env* antibodies [219]. With the intention to further develop this hypothesis, Richardson and co-workers undertook an evaluation of the effect of vaccination with the FIV *env* gene on the development of infection in cats after challenge [220]. Three groups of cats were thereby immunized using plasmid DNAs expressing either the wild-type envelope or two envelopes bearing mutations in the PID of the TM glycoprotein. This genetic immunization elicited low or undetectable levels of antibodies directed against envelope glycoproteins, hypothetically due to the vaccination protocol used. Upon homologous challenge, determination of plasma virus load showed that the acute phase of viral infection occurred earlier in all three groups of cats immunized with FIV envelopes than in the control cats. Although the influence of antibodies could not be completely excluded, the authors found no evidence of presence of antibodies or other soluble factors capable of augmenting viral infection *in vitro*, and therefore speculate that other immune phenomena, such as cellular activation, may have caused the acceleration of infection. FIV is known to replicate more efficiently in activated cells both *in vitro* and *in vivo*, as has been shown for HIV-1, and can infect B and T lymphocytes. Specific priming of cells of T and B lineages by *env* vaccination, while insufficient for the induction of detectable levels of antibodies, may have been sufficient to render cells more susceptible to viral infection. This study opens discussion to mechanisms unrelated to enhancing antibodies, linked with acceleration of virus replication.

A recent study focused on the influence of antigenic properties of live attenuated vaccines in their protection potential against lentivirus infection. Random amino acid substitutions were introduced into the TM envelope glycoprotein of FIV, within the PID, which notably bears immunodominant B cell epitopes. Amongst a wide set of mutants, those that modified antibody specificity without abolishing infectivity *ex vivo* were selected to infect a group of spf cats. After 1 year of infection, the cats were superinfected with a heterologous intraclade primary strain of FIV. One selected mutant, designated TN92, thereby succeeded in providing a significant protection of the cats against high viral loads. The authors suggested that this protection correlated with a decrease, in TN92, of the immunogenicity of a B cell epitope potentially involved in antibody enhancement of infection, thus emphasizing the importance of PID in the induction of such antibodies [221].

Viral enhancement warrants caution in the design of antiviral vaccines. Moreover, there should be considerable concern over the use of vaccines against viruses that induce infectivity enhancing antibodies, as these vaccines could then predispose the host to persistent infection or lead to selection of «enhancable» virus types. It has been shown that antibody responses induced by subunit vaccines tend to be associated with severe disease by several retroviruses. A possible approach to the development of such vaccines against this virus family might be the induction of cellular immunity rather than antibodies. In this way, plasmid DNA and viral vector-based vaccines, as well as live attenuated vaccines, can be designed to induce strong CTL responses that avoid harmful antibody responses. Indeed, as a prerequisite to the development of vaccines against lentiviruses, we must learn which interactions between virus and host immunity determine the balance between enhancement and protection and how this balance may be displaced in favor of protection.

3.2 CpG Oligonucleotide Literature Overview

After a brief introduction on the state of research in the field regarding innate immunity and the importance of Toll-like receptors (TLRs) for the early recognition of various pathogens, the following chapter will give an overview on important discovered facts concerning CpG oligonucleotides, the knowledge acquired on their immunological effects, and progress involving their use in different disease settings. The medical potential of CpG DNA has attracted high interest from scientists worldwide, and hundreds of studies aiming at the further understanding, characterization and manipulation of their effects on the host immune system have been accomplished in the last 20 years. Among the numerous published projects involving CpG ODN, a narrow selection was chosen in order to support the facts described below.

3.2.1 Insight on Innate Immunity and Toll-like Receptors

All living beings are constantly exposed to microorganisms that are present in the environment, and have consequently developed over time a means to cope with invasion of microbial pathogens in the body. The vertebrate immune system utilizes two general strategies to combat infectious diseases: innate and acquired immunity. The latter represents a specific but rather slow process, in which clonally distributed T and B cells, expressing highly specific receptors that mediate pathogen recognition, need time to proliferate after antigen contact. This highly sophisticated system of antigen detection is found only in vertebrates and has been the subject of considerable research. Initially thought to be relatively non-specific, innate immunity had, in contrast, attracted far less attention. However, the organism's first line of defence reacts immediately in presence of antigen and its considerable contribution to the activation of more specific subsequent immune responses, particularly Th1 cellular responses, must not be underestimated [222]. Not only innate immunity discriminates between self and foreign antigens, but its ability to induce rapid production of highly potent cytokines, chemokines and polyreactive antibodies allows reaction to a wide variety of pathogens with a greater degree of specificity than previously thought. Thus, scientists have shown increasing interest over the past years in understanding the complex unfolding of innate immune mechanisms, and findings have altered global ideas about the pathogenesis and treatment of cancers, as well as infectious, immune and allergic diseases.

According to a concept elaborated by Janeway and co-workers [223], early pathogen recognition mechanisms within the innate immune system relies on its ability to recognize pathogen-associated molecular patterns (PAMPs), which comprise essential and evolutionarily conserved microbial structures such as bacterial cell wall components, as well as various viral, fungal and parasite structures. The fact that these features are essential for the survival of the pathogen ensures that no mutation can arise that would avoid their recognition by the host's immune system. The detection of PAMPs relies, to great extent, on a limited set of pattern recognition receptors (PRRs), among which a small family, known as the Toll-like receptors (TLRs), has proven to allow induction of antimicrobial effector mechanisms, and thus play a crucial role in early host defence against invading pathogens [224]. Relevance of the TLR family in innate immunity was revealed in 1996, when a key Drosophila protein, *Toll*, was shown to be required not only in embryonic development for flies, but also in order to provoke an effective immune response against the fungus *Aspergillus fumigatus* [225]. To date, 11 Toll-like receptors (TLR1-TLR11) in human and 12 in mice have been identified. The TLRs are type I transmembrane proteins expressed primarily in immune cells responsible for the first line of defence, including macrophages, dendritic cells, mucosal epithelial cells, neutrophils and dermal endothelial cells [226]. Due to considerable homology in the cytoplasmic region, they are members of a larger family that includes the interleukin-1 receptors (IL-1Rs). TLRs and IL-1Rs have a conserved region of about 200 amino acids in their cytoplasmatic tails, known as the TLR/IL-1R (TIR) domain [227]. Within the TIR domain, the regions of homology comprise three conserved boxes, which are crucial for signalling. The signal transduction pathway activated by the TIR superfamily is of great importance in evolution because it is highly conserved in plants, drosophila, nematodes, avian and mammals [228]. Briefly, after ligand binding, TLRs/IL-1Rs dimerize and undergo conformational change required for the recruitment of downstream signalling molecules. These include the adaptor molecule myeloid differentiation primary response protein 88 (MyD88), IL-1R-associated kinases (IRAKs), transforming growth factor-β (TGF-β)-activated kinase 1 (TAK1), TAK1-binding protein 1 (TAB1), TAB2 and tumor necrosis factor (TNF)-receptor-associated factor 6 (TRAF6) [229]. Figure 7 represents an example of the signals instigated after activation of a Toll-like receptor. The TIR signalling cascade eventually leads to activation of several transcription factors including nuclear transcription factor κB (NFκB) and activating protein 1 (AP1), thus allowing expression of their target genes. In this way, presence of PAMPs on invading organisms initiates a downstream signal conferring to production of reactive oxygen species (ROS), inflammatory cytokines, interferons and chemokines, which all represent protective measures to defend hosts. However, it is important to keep in mind that hyper or hypo-responsiveness of TLRs or uncontrolled and improper signalling from these receptors could have serious consequences in hosts. Indeed, given the role of TLRs in the induction of such strong inflammation, the plausibility that improper regulations of the signalling pathway mediated by these proteins may also be involved in multiple inflammatory diseases such as sepsis and cancer should not be underestimated.

Remarkably, despite high conservation in extracellular regions, different TLRs can recognize several structurally unrelated ligands. The subcellular location of different TLRs correlates to some extent with the molecular patterns of their ligands. Thus, TLR1, TLR2, and TLR4 are located on the cell surface and are recruited to phagosomes after activation by their respective ligands. In contrast, TLR3, TLR7, and TLR9, all of which are involved in the recognition of nucleic acid-like structures, are not expressed on the cell surface [230]. Furthermore, it seems that TLRs are not restricted to microbial PAMPs but recognize a wide variety of ligands. Thus, they play an essential role in non-infectious sterile inflammation and can detect ligands from damaged cells such as β-defensins and oxidized lipids, among other

Literature

endogenous componds [231]. More importantly, low molecular weight synthetic molecules, such as imidazoquinolines or polyriboinosinic–polyribocytidylic acid (poly IC), which have no obvious structural similarity to PAMPs, can successfully activate signal transduction mediated by TLRs. Natural ligands have been identified for most of the TLRs known [232, 233]. Altogether, these facts support the hypothesis that synthetic blocking of the TLR pathway in inflammation settings, or enhancement of the TLR signal in immune unresponsive diseases might offer new ways of therapeutic intervention.

In conclusion, TLR identification is among the most important and fundamental discoveries in microbial pathogenesis. Today, innate immunity is increasingly recognized as the central defence system because its mechanisms also empower the adaptive immune responses. Moreover, possibility of TLR triggering with purified compounds or synthetic ligands represents a powerful means to modulate innate as well as adaptive immune responses. Many pharmaceutical companies are involved in synthesizing small molecules that can serve as TLR antagonists or agonists. Since innate immune response is not pathogen-specific, any intervention in the TLR pathway could have a broad spectrum of use. *Toll* opens an exciting new perspective in drug development, which will continue to significantly improve the quality of human and animal life in a close future.

3.2.2 Definition of CpGs and Natural Occurence

The term CpG designates a pair of nucleotides, cytosine (C) and guanine (G), appearing successively in this order along one DNA strand, separated only by a phosphate molecule (p). Within most eukaryotic DNA, CpG dinucleotides are encountered far less frequently than the expected ratio of 1:16. It seems this CpG suppression in vertebrate gemones is related to undergoing of excessive methylation in these dinucleotides of the cytosine residues at position C5. An analysis of nearest neighbour dinucleotide frequencies together with the level of DNA methylation in animals indeed strongly indicated that 5-methylcytosine (5mC) tends to mutate abnormally frequently to thymine (T) [234].

In contrast, unmethylated CpG dinucleotides are abundant in all bacterial as well as in some viral [235] and invertebrate eukaryotic genomes (e.g. drosophila) [236]. Estimations indicate a 100-fold lower presence of CpG motifs in vertebrate than in microbial DNA [237]. This critical difference in frequency and methylation of CpG sequences in the genomes of vertebrates and microorganisms is the origin of recognition of CpG motifs by the vertebrate immune system. Since CpG sequences are not only far more frequent, but also non-methylated in genomes of bacterial pathogens, the number of «free», or available motifs in prokaryotic DNA exceeds that in vertebrate DNA. These «free» CpG motifs are sensed by cells of the immune system of vertebrates and subsequently signal infectious danger to the host. The rare CpG motifs in vertebrate genomes seem not to be accessible for immune recognition, probably due to the methylation of cytosine residues.

The immune system of fish, birds and mammals all recognize and respond to CpG DNA. The evolutionary conservation of CpG recognition over millions of years strongly suggests that the immune response elicited by these motifs contributes to host survival. Further characterization of these responses thus represents great hope for future discovery of preventive and therapeutic possibilities for various diseases.

3.2.3 Uptake Mechanisms and Signal Transduction

One of the most fundamental steps in defining the molecular mechanism of action of CpG DNA was identifying its receptor. In 2000, Hemmi and co-workers from Akira's group noticed stunning similarities between the signalling mechanisms observed after cellular CpG DNA activation and the previously described signalling cascade linked to Toll-like receptors [238]. They were able to identify TLR9, a new Toll-like receptor, capable of distinguishing bacterial DNA from self-DNA. In their study, mice genetically deficient in this molecule lacked CpG-induced immune activation, indicating that expression of TLR9 is both necessary and sufficient for signal transduction after CpG administration. Chuang and Ulevitch further characterized TLR9 as a type I membrane protein preferentially expressed in immune cell rich tissues, such as spleen, lymph node, bone marrow and peripheral blood leukocytes [239]. Similarly to the previously described TLR7 and TLR8, the newly described TLR9 was shown to stimulate an NFkB signalling pathway, supporting the involvement of all these receptors in cellular responses to stimuli which activate innate immunity.

These observations were rapidly extended, by Takeshita and colleagues, to human cells, also indicating human TLR9 expression as a prerequisite for CpG ODNs responsiveness [240]. Interestingly, Bauer and co-workers further suggested that evolutionary divergence between TLR9 molecules underlies species-specific differences in the recognition of bacterial DNA. Transfection of human embryonic kidney 293 cells to express the mouse TLR9 protein rendered them optimally responsive to a different CpG motif than 293 cells transfected to express the human TLR9 analogue. The optimal CpG motif for human TLR9 activation was GTCGTT, whereas the optimal murine sequence was GACGTT [241].

Hemmi, Takeshita and Bauer all suggested presence of both TLR9 and CpG DNA in the same endocytic vesicles and hypothesized interaction and start of signal transduction in endosomes. It had indeed already been previously demonstrated that in living and unfixed cells, ODNs tend to localize in endosomes. It seems that the acidic and reducing conditions present in this intracellular compartment lead to degradation of double-stranded DNA into multiple single-stranded CpG motif- containing regions that subsequently interact directly with TLR9 [230, 242]. Compounds that block endosomal acidification, such as bafilomycin and chloroquine, inhibit CpG DNA-driven signalling [243]. An *in vitro* experiment also demonstrated that TLR9 interacted with CpG DNA more strongly at the acidic pH (6.5 or 5.5) condition [244]. However, the requirement of acidic pH in CpG recognition has recently been challenged by a study showing that a chimeric TLR9 localized to the cell surface is still capable of responding to CpG DNA [245].

The authors suggest that the expression of TLR9 in intracellular compartments is important for preventing recognition of self DNA. Therefore, although endosomal uptake is widely recognized as a prerequisite for CpG-specific responses as well as the initiation site for signal transduction through TLR9, further studies are required to clarify the role of endosomal acidification in CpG DNA recognition.

Over the years, discussions about cellular uptake of ODNs have been quite controversial. In general, it is now accepted that cellular uptake is a crucial first step in CpG-arbitrated effects and that, although probably receptor-mediated, it is not specific to CpG motifs, but more affected by the structure of the ODNs. In this way, uptake rates were demonstrated to be severely affected by backbone modifications (see 3.2.2.4) of the applied CpG sequences. It seems indeed that synthetically modified CpG ODN are taken up much more efficiently than their natural analogues [246]. Additionally, strings of guanosines (polyG) were able to increase the uptake of CpG motifs [247]. Although uptake mechanisms remain unclear, this step seems to be modifiable by different means and should not be underestimated as an important restriction point in CpG signalling.

TLR9 activation results in the induction of a classical TLR signalling cascade involving MyD88, IRAK, TRAF6, and finally resulting in activation of MAP kinases and NFκB (see figure 7) [248]. These transcription factors initiate production of type I IFN, very important antiviral molecules (see 3.2.4.3), in addition to a conserved program of pro-inflammatory signals. In contrast to TLR3 and TLR4, which have been described to use additional adaptor proteins apart from MyD88, signal transduction in response to TLR9 is critically dependent on MyD88 [249]. Although similar transducer proteins are used by various TLRs, the gene profiles of recognized PAMPs differ [250]. Thus, CpG DNA activates not only the expression of certain genes also triggered by other TLR ligands, but also a set of «CpG-specific» genes. Among the latter, importance must be attributed to the high capacity of CpG to induce production of Il-12, which plays a crucial role in the immunological properties of CpG ODN.

Literature

At this point, it must be noted that natural or synthetic structural modifications of ODNs as well as host species in which they are applied greatly influence CpG signalling at different stages of the signal transduction cascade. These facts must also imperatively be kept in mind when analyzing immunological aspects of CpG DNA (see below: 3.2.4).

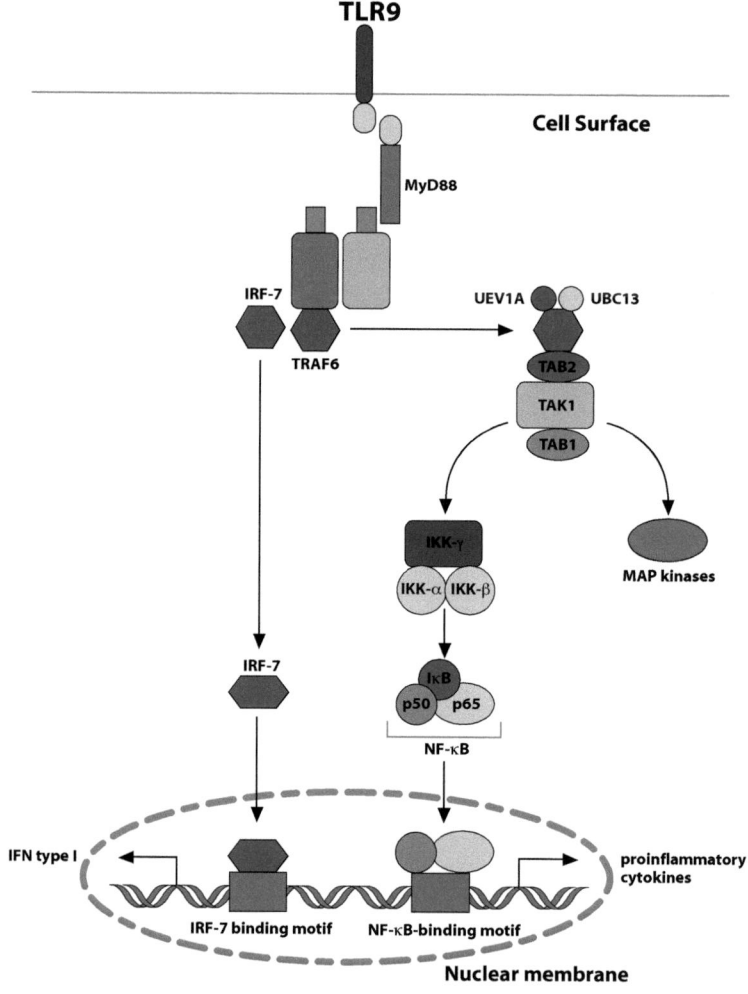

Figure 7: Signalling cascade following trigger of the TLR9

3.2.4 Immunological Effects of CpGs

Several different observations have led to the recognition of immunostimulatory DNA motifs. In the 1970s already, the successful treatment of cancer with *Mycobacterium bovis* in experimental animal models and in humans had attracted great attention [251]. It took another 10 years before another group identified a DNA-rich fraction, which they termed MY-1, as the active compound in *M. bovis* allowing tumour regression [252]. MY-1 was later shown to additionally induce IFN secretion from spleen cells and activate NK cells [253]. Moreover, all antiviral and antitumor properties of MY-1 were sensitive to DNase. Randomly selecting and testing DNA sequences of mycobacteria, Yamamoto and co-workers successfully identified a 45-mer ODN that was able to activate IFN secretion and NK cell activation [254]. Interestingly, further characterization of this ODN revealed that it contained a palindromic sequence motif with a central C-G dinucleotide, which appeared to be essential for the effects observed.

More hints to the immunological potential of DNA arose from the findings of Messina and colleagues [255]. This group was first to support the assumption that DNA from various species differed in their immunological activity. They showed that bacterial DNA was mitogenic for B lymphocytes *in vitro*, while DNA from vertebrates was not. Moreover, they demonstrated that methylation of cytosine residues of bacterial DNA completely abolished mitogenicity, indicating a DNA-sequence-dependent activity on B cells.

Unexpected immunostimulatory effects observed in the course of studies utilizing antisense ODNs also attracted particular attention. Initially, antisense ODNs were introduced in the cells to specifically prevent translation of target mRNA and, as a consequence, expression of the corresponding gene product. Several investigators observed however a sequence-specific B cell proliferation and upregulation of MHC molecules on these cells. With the aim to define more precisely the motifs inducing such effects, Krieg et al. reported that short (approximately 20 bp long) ODNs exhibited profound stimulation of B cell activity, provided they contained a central

Literature

CpG motif flanked at the 5'end by 2 purines and at the 3'end by 2 pyrimidines [256]. Moreover, both reversal of the central CpG dinucleotide to a GpC dinucleotide and methylation of the CpG dinucleotide completely abrogated mitogenic effect of the ODN on B cells.

These different lines of observations shed light on the recognition of prokaryotic DNA by the vertebrate immune system as well as on its potential to induce important immunological responses in the host. Researchers have then concentrated efforts in understanding the unfolding of these responses and thus uncovered mechanisms which have allowed satisfying use of CpG motifs in various disease settings. The following chapter discusses the known immunological effects of CpG DNA.

3.2.4.1 Cellular Immunology of CpG DNA

CpG motif recognition by the immune system of vertebrates results in a direct stimulation of TLR9 expressing cell types, mainly including dendritic cells (DCs) and B cells. Activated DCs subsequently mature and produce signals allowing stimulation of macrophages and monocytes, increased activation of NK cells, and maturation of naive T cells to a Th1 phenotype. Since activated T cells have the potential to induce more specific responses to various antigens, CpG also indirectly improve the host's ability to mount a subsequent adaptive immune response (see figure 8).

CpG ODNs thus not only strengthen early immune responses, but additionally prepare the adaptive immune components to possible pathogen contact and reaction with a Th1-directed response, creating an interesting link between innate and adaptive immunity. The more detailed understanding of these immunomodulatory properties was crucial to the increasing popularity of CpG ODNs observed over the years in research and pharmaceutical fields.

3.2.4.1.1 B Cells

Krieg and co-workers were the first to describe in 1995, that bacterial DNA and ODNs containing CpG motifs could induce murine B cells to proliferate and secrete immunoglobulins *in vitro* and *in vivo* [256]. Ever since, experiments including various species have equally shown extraordinarily strong mitogen effects of CpG ODNs for B cells from essentially all vertebrates, including humans [257], non-human primates [258], cows [259], as well as most of all common farm and pet companion animals [260]. CpG ODNs not only enhance proliferation of B cells, but activate their secretion of cytokines (mostly IL-6) and immunglobulins as well as the expression on their surface of increased levels of Fcγ receptor and co-stimulatory molecules, such as class II MHC, CD80 and CD86. Yi and colleagues demonstrated that CpG ODN rapidly induce B cells to enter the G1 phase of the cell cycle and secrete IL-6 [261]. *In vitro* treatment of a B cell line with CpG DNA led to an increase in the transcriptional activity of the IL-6 promoter. Moreover, within 30 minutes after CpG DNA stimulation *in vivo*, IL-6 mRNA levels were increased in murine liver, spleen, and thymus cells. Serum IL-6 protein was markedly increased within 1 hour of stimulation. Additionally, the CpG-induced IL-6 expression was shown to be required for subsequent B cell secretion of IgM.

Activation of mature peripheral B cells by CpG ODNs was shown to be enhanced by simultaneous signals delivered through the B cell antigen receptor (BCR). Indeed, Krieg and co-workers had already indicated strong synergy of low concentrations of CpG with BCR-triggering signals, leading to an approximate 10-fold increase in B cell proliferation and antigen-specific immuoglobulin (Ig) and IL-6 secretion [256]. Thus, in the presence of antigen, CpG ODNs have an even greater immunologic potential on B cells, and allow under such conditions, the passage to a more specific type of immune response.

Finally, Yi and co-workers suggested that CpG-containing ODN motifs provide signals not only for cell cycle entry, but also for cellular survival [262]. Specific

Literature

and/or cooperative interactions of multiple genes, upregulated by the presence of CpG, conferred to the rescue of a murine B lymphoma cell line from anti-IgM-induced cell cycle arrest and apoptosis. In another experiment, the same group demonstrated that treatment of isolated murine B cells with CpG reversed their tendency to spontaneous apoptosis in a sequence-specific fashion [263]. Indeed, reversal of the CG to GC as well as methylation of the central cytosine both significantly decreased this activity. CpG DNA has also been reported to protect B cells against Fas-mediated apoptosis by downregulating Fas expression on CD40-stimulated B cells [264].

3.2.4.1.2 Dendritic Cells

Dentritic cells play a central role in the effect of CpG on the immune system. Their function as antigen-presenting cells (APCs) as well as their ability to produce a wide variety of pro-inflammatory cytokines render them the important intermediate signals to specific T cell immunity. Thus, they create the link between the innate and the acquired immune system and influence the balance between Th1 and Th2 immune responses. Studies on the effects of CpG motifs on DCs have mainly been carried out on mouse and human cellular models. Sparwasser and colleagues were the first to demonstrate that bacterial DNA or synthetic CpG ODNs cause simultaneous maturation of immature murine DCs, upregulating of MHC class II, CD40 and CD86 molecules on their surface, and activation of mature murine DCs to produce large amounts of cytokines, such as IL-12, IL-6 and TNF-α [265]. Similarly, Hartmann et al. showed that CpG ODNs alone were superior to GMCSF in promoting survival and maturation (CD83 expression) as well as expression of class II MHC and the co-stimulatory molecules CD40, CD54, and CD86 of human DCs [266].

With the identification of TLR9 as cellular receptor for CpG recognition, it was rapidly determined that individual subsets of murine and human DCs express different TLR molecules which enable them to respond to distinct pathogens and thus induce diverse patterns of immune reactions [267]. Thus, among human DCs, a subset termed «plasmacytoid» (pDC), due to its microscopic appearance similar to that of plasmablasts, strongly expresses TLR9. Instead, myeloid lineages of DCs express mainly other TLRs, rendering them susceptible to other sets of pathogen molecules, including Lipopolysaccharide (LPS) for example.

In humans, only the pDC subset has so far clearly demonstrated direct activation by CpG DNA [268]. After stimulation with CpG, these DCs showed an increased ability to induce proliferation of naive allogeneic CD4+ T cells. They were also shown to express CCR7, which mediates their homing to lymph nodes. Additionally, interactions of DCs with NK cells have been reported in mice [253], as well as in humans [269]. In the latter study, pDCs enhanced NK cell activity in a cytotoxicity assay, both with and without direct contact between DCs and NK cells (further details under 3.2.4.1.4). Finally, it must be mentioned that pDC represent the primary source of type I IFN, a potent driver of Th1 development and cell-mediated antiviral immunity (see 3.2.4.3).

Subcutaneous administration of CpG DNA also leads to *in vivo* stimulation of skin Langerhans cells to upregulate co-stimulatory molecules and produce IL-12, as well as to undergo morphologic changes and migration [270].

In summary, CpG DNA induces maturation of human and murine DCs to professional APCs, which in turn secrete a series of pro-inflammatory and Th1 type cytokines, favouring maturation of CD4 cells to the Th1 subtype. CpG also activates migration of DCs, thus augmenting their rapidity and potential of effect.

3.2.4.1.3 Monocytes and Macrophages

The effects of CpG ODNs on monocyte/macrophage lineages of humans and mice have been compared. Interestingly, purified human monocytes do not express TLR9 and are, as a result, not activated by CPG ODNs. Nevertheless, CpG DNA treatment of human PBMCs or whole blood secondarily activates the monocytes to express CD40 and CD69, and to produce IL-6 and TNF-α. These findings have been mainly attributed to effects of backbones used in synthetic CpG ODN production (see 3.2.6) [271]. In contast, in murine monocytes/macrophages, CpG DNA has been shown to trigger induction of nuclear translocation of NFκB, accumulate TNF-α mRNA and release large amounts of TNF-α [272]. These findings suggest a species-specific response of certain cell types to CpG ODNs. Further details to species specificity of CpG ODNs are described in section 3.2.5.

3.2.4.1.4 Natural Killer Cells

Both murine and human NK cells lack TLR9 expression and are thus not directly stimulated by CpG ODNs. Since the initial observation that mycobacterial DNA activates murine NK cells to produce IFN-γ and to have lytic activity [273], many efforts have been concentrated on elucidating the mechanism that generates these findings. It remained controversial for a long time, whether it was the structure of the ODN or the presence of CpG sequences that induced the observed effects on NK cells [274]. An interesting study from Ballas and colleagues showed the explicit requirement of an unmethylated CpG motif included in short ODN sequences for the induction of NK cell lytic activity *in vitro* in both human and murine lymphocytes as well as *in vivo*, in mice [275]. Furthermore, in experiments designed to determine the cellular and cytokine settings necessary for CpG-mediated NK cell stimulation, the same group revealed that ODNs could not augment the activity of highly purified NK cells, and that increased NK cell activity depended on the presence of adherent cells or CpG-conditioned supernatants, which contain IL-12, TNF-γ, and type I IFN.

A series of subsequent studies permitted the further characterization of the link between CpG-related activation and effector mechanisms of NK cells. Cowdery and co-workers showed that bacterial DNA induces *in vivo* release of IFN-γ and identified NK cells by surface phenotyping as the main IFN-γ producing cells [276]. Later on, dependence of IFN-γ production in PBMCs on CpG ODN-induced IFN-α/β was demonstrated by IFN-α/β-blocking antibodies [277]. In this study, the potency of CpG ODNs to stimulate IFN-α correlated with their ability to stimulate NK cell lytic activity. Recently, the responsibility for the stimulation of NK cells with CpG ODNs has been attributed to pDCs. Indeed, partial activation of NK cells was mediated by pDC-derived IFN-α, whereas full activation of NK cells, indicated by IFN-γ production, required cell-to-cell contact of pDCs and NK cells in addition to IFN-α[278]. Importantly, as mentioned above (3.2.4.1.2), interactions between pDCs with NK cells had been reported earlier in mice as well as in humans [253] [269].

The role of pDCs as intermediate signals for NK cell stimulation through CpG has recently been extended, as another CpG-induced pDC factor, TNF-α, was shown to participate in the production of IFN-γ by NK cells in an additive fashion. Nevertheless, this particular activity of TNF-α required the presence of a co-factor such as IFN-α [279].

3.2.4.1.5 T Cells

Due to their lack of TLR9 expression, it is widely accepted that T cells cannot be directly stimulated by CpG ODNs [280]. Thus, activation of T cells by CpG ODNs was rapidly linked to an indirect effect involving professional APCs, such as DCs. Three mechanisms of indirect CpG-related stimulation of T cells by DCs are known to date. First, CpG ODNs have been reported to upregulate co-stimulatory molecules and MHC class II molecules on DCs (see 3.2.4.1.2). Such molecules are critical for the recognition of antigens by T cells and their enhanced expression on DCs can result in a more efficient antigen presentation to CD4+ T cells. Furthermore, CpG ODNs stimulate IL-12 secretion by DCs, which is the main factor triggering IFN-γ production by CD4+ T cells. Finally, CpG ODNs induce secretion of IL-6 by DCs via TLR9-mediated signalling. The secreted IL-6 blocks at least in part the suppressive effect of CD4+CD25+ regulatory T cells (Treg) on CTL [281], allowing full activation of pathogen specific CD8+ T cells. Thus, a block of Treg cell functions by CpG ODN-stimulated DCs might provide new means to augment specific immunity in infectious diseases. In conclusion, both the molecular modifications and the specific cytokine secretion of DCs augment pathogen-specific T cell responses and IFN-γ release during an ongoing bacterial infection, or following CpG ODN stimulation.

3.2.4.1.6 Neutrophils

Neither enhanced oxidative burst nor increased expression of activation markers has been identified on the neutrophil population after CpG treatment *in vitro*. However, Weighardt et al. demonstrated that subsequent to administration of CpG ODNs *in vivo*, mice showed substantially increased resistance against acute polymicrobial sepsis, together with a strongly enhanced accumulation of neutrophils at the primary site of infection [282]. Additionally, neutrophils of CpG ODN-treated mice exhibited an upregulation of phagocytic receptors, an increased phagocytic activity, and an elevated production of reactive oxygen metabolites. Thus, CpG DNA does not appear to activate neutrophils directly, but may improve their ability to provide effective host defence.

3.2.4.2 Creation of Th1-like Cytokine Milieu

The activation of immune cells by CpG DNA initiates a complex network of cell-cell interactions and cytokine production cascades that result in an overall enhancement of immune functions in an antigen-independent manner. This immune stimulation is strongly Th1-directed, since these defence mechanisms are originally optimized for protection against intracellular pathogens. Put together, the cellular mechanisms described above induce production of high amounts of IL-12 and IFN-γ, which are considered key factors for the development of Th1-deviated reactivity. They directly or indirectly promote proliferation and differentiation of Th1 cells, activate phagocytic and NK cells against microbial infections, and are required for the development of CTL-mediated immunity against viral infections or malignant cells. Moreover, IFN-γ enhances Th1 antibody production by B cells by inducing IgM to Ig2a isotype switching. Klinman and colleagues were the first to describe the ability of CpG motifs to induce Th1 and pro-inflammatory cytokine production *in vitro* and *in vivo* [283]. Systemic injection of CpG DNA was thereby shown to create a systemic Th1-like response. Likewise, local injection of CpG subcutaneously into the footpad of mice induced IL-12 and IFN-γ production in the draining lymph nodes and lymphadenopathy that peaked at 7-10 days post-treatment. DCs became a more prominent population in the lymph nodes and exhibited an activated phenotype with increased expression of co-stimulatory molecules [284]. Intradermal or intranasal delivery of CpG DNA also resulted in a localized state of Th1 predisposition [285]. The possibility to induce this Th1 environment is of great interest in vaccination and treatment of diseases that are characterized by Th2 immune deviations, which appear insufficient in clearing the affection.

3.2.4.3 Production of Interferon-α

Probably the most important antiviral property of CpG ODNs resides in their potential to stimulate the production of high amounts of IFN-α by the pDCs, also known as interferon-producing cells [286]. IFN-α prevents viral dissemination by both directly impairing proper viral replication and promoting the functions of various cell populations responsible for the first response to invading organisms. Indeed, this type I IFN has been shown to considerably enhance NK cell cytolytic activity, promote differenciation, maturation and immunostimulatory functions of monocytes and DCs [287], induce B cells to produce immunoglobulin [288], and induce Th1 differentiation of T cells [289]. Moreover, IFN-α effectively induces the synthesis of various cellular proteins, including enzymes, signalling proteins, antigen presenting proteins and transcription factors, which initiate its antiviral properties. IFN-α effector proteins possess the ability to interfere with several steps of the virus cycle, thus preventing virus from replicating in yet uninfected cells. In summary, INF-α plays a key role in the mounting of a global «antiviral state» comprising potent defence mechanisms against viral infection.

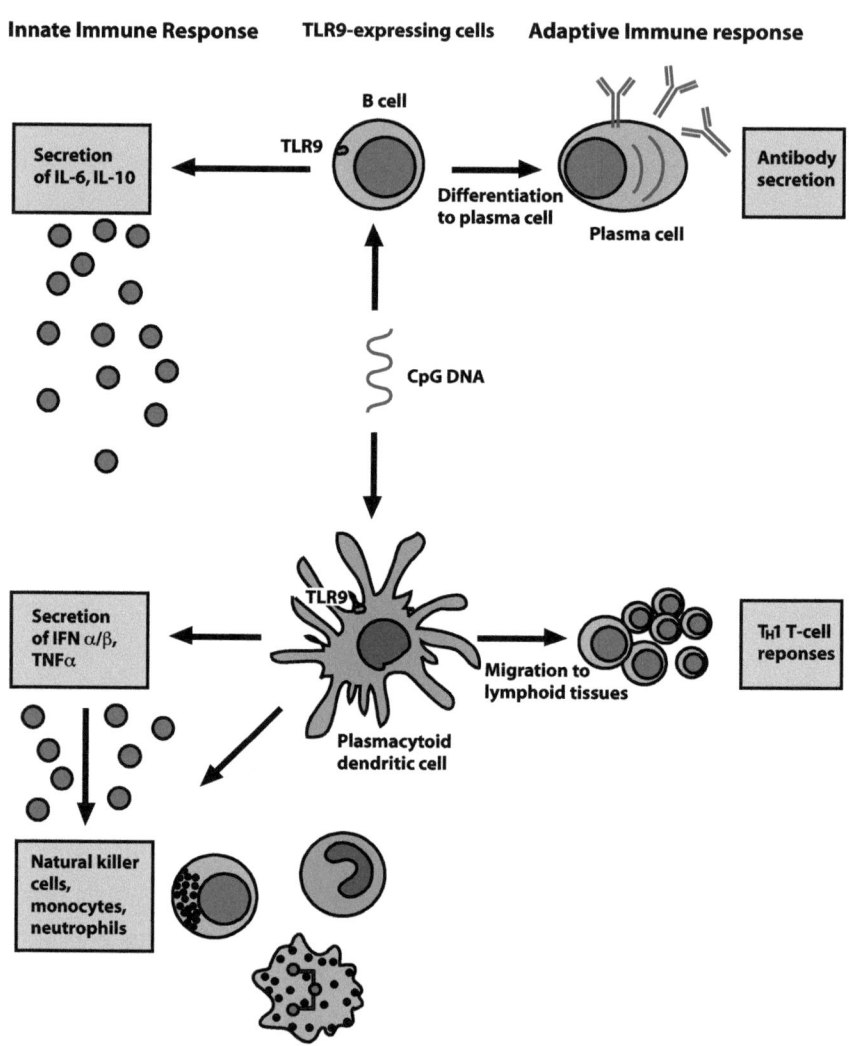

Figure 8: The immunostimulatory effects of TLR9 activation in pDCs and B cells

Immune System	Humoral Effects	Cellular Effects
Innate Immunity	IFN-α secretion	
	Secretion of IFN-inducible chemokines and cytokines	NK cell lytic activity
	Secretion of pro-inflammatory cytokines (IL-6, TNF-α)	Neutrophil activation, migration and bacterial uptake
	Secretion of anti-inflammatory cytokines (IL-10, IL-1RA)	
Adaptive Immunity	Induction of IgG isotype switching and antibody secretion	Differentiation of Th1 cells
	Suppression of IgE antibody production	Enhanced cross-priming
		Increased CTL activity

Table 8: Breadth of the CpG-induced immune response

3.2.5 Species Specificity in CpG DNA Recognition

Early studies proposed a degree of species specificity in the recognition of CpG motifs. It was thought that the precise sequence motifs (unmethylated CpG dinucleotides and flanking regions) optimal for stimulating immune cells from one species differed from those optimal for another species due to evolutionary divergences in TLR9 molecules. In this way, the TLR9 molecules in mice were shown to differ from those in humans by 24% at the amino acid level, and the terms mouse (GACGTT) and human (GTCGTT) CpG motifs were adopted [241]. Indeed, the optimal murine CpG motif was shown to have little, if any stimulatory activity on cells from humans, chimpanzees and rhesus monkeys [258].

It is crucial to point out however, that initial experiments were restricted to murine and human cells. Several studies examining effects of different CpG motifs in a larger variety of animals have indicated that the GTCGTT sequence is optimal for stimulation of lymphocyte proliferation in many different species. Verthelyi and Klinman showed that PBMCs from humans, macaques, chimpanzees and orangutans respond to the same class of CpG ODN [290]. Moreover, analysis of CpG DNA efficacy in various veterinary and laboratory species, including cattle, sheep, goats, horses, dogs, cats and chicken, demonstrated that in all species tested, the GTCGTT motif seemed to have stimulatory potential [260]. Not only there appeared to be little evidence of divergence in terms of actual motif recognition, but other requirements for ODN stimulation, such as the nature and degree of spacing between motifs or requirements for particular 5' bases preceding the motifs, were also similar among the species tested. In addition, there was no apparent variation in the stimulatory effect of ODNs based on age, gender, or breed. Interestingly, the only apparent exceptions in recognition and immune stimulation potential of particular CpG-containing sequences seemed to be laboratory mice and rabbits. The authors suggest that inbreeding of the animals used for research purposes may have had an important impact on response to CpGs. A subsequent study in dogs and cats [291] has confirmed evidence of cross-species activity of the GTCGTT motif. Altogether, these observations indicate that CpG motif recognition remains an ancient evolutionary adaptation in a broad variety of species, more highly conserved than previously thought.

The cell populations that express TLR9 might differ between species. Again, major differences have been mostly identified between mice and primates. Thus, murine immune cells of the myeloid lineage (including monocytes, macrophages, and myeloid DCs) express TLR9 and respond to CpG stimulation, whereas in humans, these cell types generally do not express TLR9 and cannot be directly activated by CpG ODNs.

Since studies that are designed to examine the therapeutic potential of CpG ODNs are typically initiated in mice, it appears crucial to ascertain the *in vivo* potential for the selected ODNs in the target species. Although activation of both murine B and NK cells *in vitro* are considered excellent predictors of cross-species *in vivo* activity [258], species-specific leukocyte proliferation assays have shown to be a more reliable predictive indicator of the *in vivo* potential of an ODN, and should be used to screen ODNs for biologic activity in different species. Since sequence, number, and spacing of individual CpG motifs contribute to the immunostimulatory activity of a CpG ODN, it is important that broad panels of ODNs be tested for their efficacy.

3.2.6 Production of Synthetic Oligonucleotides

Synthetic oligonucleotides containing CpG motifs similar to those found in bacterial DNA induce comparable immune responses. Moreover, synthetic ODNs can be produced in a sequence-specific manner, in large quantities and with high purity. These facts render synthetic immunomodulatory ODNs particularly interesting in terms of therapeutic use for many diseases. Synthesizing of effective ODNs however imperatively requires the consideration of different important variables, including stability of the compound *in vivo* and species-specific recognition of the sequence, as well as the possibility of undesired side effects. Finally, establishment of reliable assays capable of indicating *in vivo* potential is crucial.

Most of the DNA sequence-specific information on immunostimulatory DNA has been derived from the analyzes with synthetic ODNs. Natural ODNs containing phosphodiester linkages (pODNs) are rapidly degraded *in vivo* and *in vitro* by the action of nucleases. Moreover, nuclease activities seem to be higher in human than in mouse cells, with the result that pODNs can appear non-stimulatory unless they are administered repeatedly. In order to stabilize them against degradation and thus increase efficacy in immune stimulation, ODNs are often made resistant to nucleases by chemically modifying the backbone of the DNA molecule. ODNs with phosphorothioate linkages (sODNs) are thereby commonly used [246]. It has been shown that sODNs are up to 100 times more efficient than pODNs of the same sequence in eliciting CpG-dependent immune responses. However, phosphorothioate backbone modifications result in various undesired side effects. Indeed, it has been shown that such modifications can lead to a prolongation of the blood clotting time [292], acute toxicities via complement activation [293], as well as splenomegally, lymphoid follicle destruction and immunosuppression [294]. Also, due to their polyanionic property, sODNs bind non-specifically to various proteins, i.e transcription factors, and thus may affect cell signalling [295]. As a result, high concentrations of sODNs and long treatment durations should generally be avoided when using this agent *in vivo*.

Literature

Following evidence that distinct types of CpG ODNs could induce differential responses by human cells [296], at least three structurally differing classes of synthetic CpG ODNs capable of stimulating cells expressing human TLR9 have been described. K-type ODNs (also known as CpG-B) encode multiple CpG motifs on a phosphorothioate backbone, and trigger the differenciation of APCs as well as the proliferation and activation of B cells [257]. D-type ODNs (also known as CpG-A) are constructed using a mixed phosphodiester-phophorothioate backbone and contain a single hexameric purine-pyrimidine-CG-purine-pyrimidine motif flanked by self-complementary bases that have the potential to form a stem-loop structure capped at the 3'end by a poly-G tail. The poly-G tails on the individual D-type ODN molecules can interact, resulting in formation of ODN clusters. It has been demonstrated that ODNs containing a palindromic CpG motif, but lacking the poly-G tail, induce reduced immune activation. D-type ODNs directly induce the secretion of IFN-α from pDCs, which supports the subsequent maturation of APCs [277]. Finally, C-type ODNs were designed to combine some of the important properties of D and K type ODNs. They resemble the K-type ODNs in being composed entirely of phosphorothioate nucleotides. Commonly expressing a TCGTCG at the 5'end, and containing a K-type motif imbedded in a palindromic sequence, this class of ODN can both stimulate B cells to secrete IL-6 and pDCs to produce IFN-α. Table 9 summarizes structural characteristics and immunomodulatory activities of the differently used synthetic ODN types.

Knowledge in DNA synthesis allows for examination of various modifications and their effects on immunological activity. Ongoing studies are directed towards creating new ODN structures, varying the numbers and sequences of CpG motifs they contain, in an effort to develop ODNs that will be useful therapeutically. In addition, determining the ability of the different produced types of ODNs to regulate specific elements of the immune system allows achievement of specific therapeutic goals. Further clinical trials will lead to a more complete understanding of the potential of differently composed CpG ODNs.

ODN Type	Example	Structural Characteristics	Immunomodulatory Activity
D-Type (A-CpG)	GGTGCATCGATGCAGGGGGG	Mixed backbone, single CpG motif	APC maturation, mediated by IFN-α
		CpG flanking region forms a palindrome	Stimulation of APCs to secrete IFN-α
		Poly-G tail at 3' end	
K-Type (B-CpG)	TCCATGGACGTTCCTGAGCGTT	Phosphorothioate backbone	pDC maturation production of TNF-α
		Multiple CpG motifs (blue)	B cell proliferation and IgM and IL-6 production
		5' motif most simulatory	
C-Type	TCGTCGTTCGAACGACGTTGAT	Phosphorothioate backbone	Activates pDCs to secrete IFN-α
		Multiple CpG motifs, TCG dimer at 5' end	Stimulates B cells to produce IgM and IL-6
		CpG motif imbedded in a central palindrome	

Table 9: Classes of CpG ODN

3.2.7 Immunotherapeutic Possibilities

The immunostimulatory potential of prokaryotic DNA has attracted great interest over the years. Unmethylated CpG motifs not only stimulate a wide variety of cells responsible for the first line of host defence against pathogens, but they deviate this early response in a Th1 direction, thus reinforcing the subsequent cellular immune mechanisms. Moreover, synthetic CpG DNA analogues have proven to be easy to produce and at rather low costs, allowing extended research as well as great hope for future clinical use in both veterinary and human medical fields. To date, prophylactic and therapeutic potentials of CpG ODNs have been evaluated for various types of cancer and states of chronic allergy, as well as against bacterial, viral and parasitical diseases. Furthermore, the immunomodulatory effects of CpG DNA have led to the assessment of their possible use as adjuvants in immunization.

The next chapters describe relevant studies and important clinical trials carried out in these various settings, highlighting the importance CpG ODNs have gained over the past years in medical science.

3.2.7.1 Protection of Immunocomprimised Hosts

A considerable benefit of CpG ODNs is their ability to boost immunity in groups of individuals with reduced immune function. Indeed, there are several conditions in which the activity of the adaptive, but not the innate immune system is compromised. Common situations are immaturity of the immune system in neonates, pregnancy, and retrovirus infections.

Pregnancy is associated with a generalized suppression of the adaptive immune system, with significant decrease in cell-mediated immunity. These changes minimize the risk that the maternal immune system might reject the fetus, but simultaneously increase the mother's risk to infection. Thus, pregnant mice usually succumb rapidly to infection by 50 LD50 of *Listeria*. In contrast, pregnant mice treated with CpG ODNs generally survived such challenge. Moreover, in the absence of CpG treatment, more than a third of the fetuses became infected within a few days of challenge, with the number of infectious organisms per fetus rising significantly over time. In contrast, none of the fetuses from CpG ODN-treated mothers became infected, indicating a positive effect of the treatment on mother-to-fetus transmission of *Listeria* [297].

Retroviral infections such as FIV, SIV, and HIV induce a progressive deterioration in the number and function of the CD4+ T cells accompanied by an increase in susceptibility to opportunistic infections. However, retroviral infection does not interfere with the activity of the innate immune system until very late in the disease process. Indeed, PBMCs from retrovirus-infected primates continue to respond strongly to CpG ODN stimulation. *In vivo*, CpG ODNs designed for human use provided significant protection to rhesus macaques infected with SIV, when challenged with *Leishmania*. Parasite load was reduced 300-fold when compared with SIV-infected animals treated with control (non-CpG) ODNs [290].

Ongoing studies indicate that CpG treatment also increases the resistance of newborns and elderly to infection [298]. Altogether, these findings indicate that

CpG ODNs significantly reduce susceptibility to infection even in situations where the host's ability to mount an adaptive immune response is compromised. This reveals the great prophylactic potential of CpG treatment on a community level: Targeting susceptible individuals reduces the likelihood of pathogen transmission and therefore enhances the community's resistance to infection.

3.2.7.2 Cancer

The decreased capacity of many tumor cell types to induce an appropriate immunogenic signal often leads to an insufficient activation of the innate immune response and, therefore, to inadequate adaptive immunity resulting in failure to eliminate or control cancer. In consideration of the fact that CpG ODNs stimulate critical components of the immune system, such as pDCs, B cells, and NK cells, involved in recognition and elimination of cancer cells, their use in cancer therapy, both alone and in combination with other anti-tumor therapies, has been widely studied. In works of recent years, CpG ODNs have indicated promising anti-tumor activity in various animal models and in humans. Furthermore, the conferred anti-tumor activity was shown to be additive or synergistic when CpG ODNs were used in combination with various chemotherapies, radiation protocols, surgery, monoclonal antibodies and cancer vaccines [299, 300].

Observed anti-tumor effects of CpG ODNs depend on the route of application, on the CpG ODN class, as well as on the type of tumor. In this way, systemic monotherapy with CpG ODNs induced regression of established, highly immunogenic tumors [301]. In other tumor models however, systemic injection of CpG ODNs has been poorly effective when compared to other routes of applications, such as peritumoral injections [302, 303]. A-class CpG ODNs appear to be more effective in NK-sensitive tumor models, whereas B-class CpG ODNs indicate anti-tumor activity where a broader immune activation, including development of T cell responses is required [304].

The combination of CpG ODN-induced TLR9 stimulation with other anti-cancer therapies has indicated powerful synergistic properties. Therapy forms that kill tumor cells, such as chemotherapy or radiation, lead to the release of tumor cell bodies that can be captured by DCs. When such DCs are co-stimulated by CpG ODNs, the presentation of tumor antigens is enhanced and stronger antitumor CD4+ and CD8+ T cell activation is induced as a result. Thus, a combination of CpG ODNs with cyclophosphamide or topotecan in an orthopaedic rhabdomyosarcoma model resulted in long term survival of the sick mice even when they presented large tumors. Interestingly, neither cyclophosphamide nor CpG ODNs alone indicated an effect on the disease [305]. Similarly, CpG ODNs have shown potential to improve clinical radiotherapy. Peritumoral administration of CpG ODNs significantly delayed tumor growth in combination with single-dose radiation, whereas identical CpG ODN treatment alone indicated little or no effect at all. Moreover, in the same study, tumors treated with both CpG ODNs and radiation showed histological changes characterised by increased necrosis, heavy infiltration by host inflammatory cells and reduced tumor density [306]. CpG ODNs also activate NK cells or macrophages that lead to enhanced efficacy of antibody therapy by increasing effector cell killing of tumor cells decorated with antibody [299]. In a mouse model, injection of CpG ODNs thus significantly increased the efficacy of monoclonal antibody therapy of lymphoma [307]. These findings were linked to the enhancement of antibody-dependent cellular cytotoxicty (ADCC) which commonly greatly contributes to the efficacy of anti-tumor antibodies used in clinical cancer trials. Finally, CpG ODNs have also proven to be effective as adjuvants in tumor vaccination models. They seem to be the only adjuvants inducing anti-tumor responses capable of resulting in the elimination of large tumors [302, 308]. Compared with other reported adjuvants, they induced increased numbers of tumour antigen-specific CD4+ and CD8+ T cells, as well as increased T cell INF-γ production [309-311]. These vaccine-enhancing effects are probably due to both CpG-mediated stimulation of DCs and the generation of Th1-promoting cytokines.

Recent clinical trials in humans also indicate that CpG ODNs represent a promising agent in the treatment of various cancer types. Several phase I and II clinical studies evaluated CpG ODNs either as a monotherapy, or in combination with antibody therapy or chemotherapy, in patients with basal cell carcinoma, melanoma, cutaneous T cell lymphoma, non-Hodgkin's lymphoma, renal cell cancer, breast cancer or non-small cell lung cancer (table 10). *In vivo* activation of pDCs and NK cells, enhanced ADCC and resulting stabilization of the disease in often more than 50% of the treated patients could be demonstrated in most of the clinical studies after parenteral administration of CpG ODN. Moreover, several studies indicated measurable regressions in tumor size after only few low-dose intra-lesional injections of CpG ODNs. The immunological properties of CpG ODNs thus indicate a great potential in the cancer therapy setting for both animals and humans.

Disease	ODN	Combination Therapy	Reference
Cancer			
Non-Hodgkin's Lymphoma	CpG 7909		299, 304, 312, 313
	CpG 7909	Rituximab	299, 304, 312, 313
	ISS 1018	Rituximab	314
Breast cancer	CpG 7909	Herceptin®	299, 312, 313
Renal cell cancer	CpG 7909		312
Non-small cell lung cancer	CpG 7909	Chemotherapy	◆
Basal cell carcinoma (intralesional)	CpG 7909		313, 315
Melanoma (intralesional)	CpG 7909		313, 315
Melanoma	CpG 7909		312, 313
	CpG 7909	Chemotherapy	◆
	CpG 7909	MAGE-3	313, 315
Cutaneous T cell lymphoma	CpG 7909		316
Infectious disease			
Hepatitis B vaccination	CpG 7909	Energix-B® in alum	315, 317, 318
	ISS 1018	Energix-B®	319
Hepatitis B vaccination (HIV + patients)	CpG 7909	Energix-B® in alum	315, 320
Influenza vaccination	CpG 7909	Fluarix®	318
Hepatitis C	CpG 10101		320
Allergy			
Allergic asthma	CpG TLR9 agonist		◆
Allergic rhinitis	ISS 1018	Amb a1	321

Table 10: Recent clinical studies using CpG ODN (adapted from Vollmer 2005, [322]) ISS: immunostimulatory sequence, ◆: Coley Pharmaceutical Group 2004

3.2.7.3 Allergy

Allergic diseases result from Th2 type immune responses against otherwise harmless environmental antigens. Such responses lead to the generation of Th2 cells, which produce cytokines such as IL-4 and IL-5 and promote the differentiation of B cells into IgE-secreting cells. This IgE binds to the high affinity IgE Fc receptor on the surface of mast cells and basophils. Subsequent exposure of these cells to an allergen results in the binding of the allergen by surface IgE, cross-linking of the IgE Fc receptors, and activation followed by degranulation of the mast cells or basophils. A variety of preformed pro-inflammatory and vasoactive compounds including histamine, prostaglandins, leukotrienes, and cytokines are released during the process of degranulation, which results in a strong, undesired inflammatory response.

There has been an increasing prevalence of allergic diseases in developed countries over the last decades. The «hygiene hypothesis» has been proposed as a possible explanation for this epidemical trend in allergy: a higher degree of hygiene as well as smaller families, inducing less contact of young children to sick siblings and reduced microbial stimulation of the TLRs in early life, which could lead to a weaker Th1 reactivity and a stronger Th2 response to allergens.

For a long time, therapeutic efforts against allergic disease have been aimed at the control of the symptoms triggered by mast cell or basophil degranulation. However, preventing the initial generation of the Th2-like immune response against allergens seems to be a more fundamental approach to disease therapy. Since Th1 and Th2 immune responses are typically mutually inhibitory, the induction of a Th1-like immune response to an allergen represents a founded alternative to indirectly suppress the Th2-like reactivity. On the basis of their potent induction of Th1 responses, the immunomodulatory properties of CpG ODNs were mainly tested in asthma, a common atopic disorder affecting animals and humans. Results of a selection of studies are described below.

Literature

Numerous reports describe the protective effects of CpG DNA on acute allergic inflammation. Kline and co-workers were the first to examine the effects of CpG ODNs in a murine model of asthma. They demonstrated that systemic CpG ODN administration prevented the development of airway eosinophilia and bronchial hyperreactivity in animals sensitized to an allergen [323]. This therapeutic response was associated with a decrease in IL-4, and an increase in IFN-γ and IL-12 in the airway fluid. Broide and colleagues additionally demonstrated that CpG ODN administration via systemic or mucosal routes effectively inhibit both systemic and airway eosinophilia and that a single such treatment with CpG DNA was at least as efficacious as seven consecutive daily injections of corticosteroids [324]. Prophylactic effects of CpGs were furthermore shown to last at least 6 weeks after a single administration, indicating effective long term prevention of asthma [325].

Reversal of established eosinophilic airway inflammation is more challenging than preventing its development. Nevertheless, Kline et al. demonstrated that systemic administration of CpG DNA and allergen was effective at reversing established airway eosinophilic inflammation [326]. Mice were thereby sensitized to ovalbulmin (OVA), and then challenged repeatedly by inhalation of the same antigen. In these animal models, significant airway eosinophilia developed within 48 hours of the first challenge, increased with additional challenges, and persisted over several weeks, thus allowing the assumption of established OVA-induced airway disease. After a course of immunotherapy using low doses of OVA, in the presence or absence of CpG ODNs, mice that had been treated with the combination of CpG ODNs and OVA were significantly protected against antigen-induced eosinophilic airway inflammation.

Repeated episodes of acute disease or chronic state of inflammation may lead to development of irreversible airway alterations collectively referred to as airway 'remodelling'. These changes have important functional consequences, including loss of distensibility of asthmatic airways, permanent airflow obstruction, and bronchial hyperreactivity, all of which persist even in the absence of further exposure to antigens. Effects of CpG ODNs on airway 'remodelling' have also been examined

[327]. For this study, a murine model of chronic asthma was created, in which OVA-sensitized mice were subjected to repeated inhalational exposure to OVA aerosol three times weekly for 6 weeks. These mice developed significant subepithelial fibrosis and goblet cell hyperplasia/metaplasia in association with chronic airway hyperreactivity. In contrast, mice that were treated with CpG DNA at the time of sensitization had significantly fewer features of airway remodelling. These results suggest that CpG ODNs associated with a specific antigen may not only be effective in reversing established airway disease, but may also prevent chronic inflammatory structural changes in the airways seen in chronic asthma.

Early human trials of CpG ODNs for atopic disorders have been promising. The immunodominant allergen from ragweed pollen, Amb a1, linked to a CpG ODN (Amb a1/immunostimulatory DNA conjugate, AIC), induces a Th1 response in PBMCs of patients allergic to ragweed, rather than the Th2 response that follows stimulation with Amb a1 alone. Thus, when subjects allergic to ragweed were treated out of season with escalating doses of AIC, they demonstrated reductions in *ex vivo* ragweed-specific Th2 responses as well as transient increases in IFN-γ [328]. In a separate study, six escalating doses of immunotherapy with AIC, administered over a short period of time, only moderately suppressed allergy symptoms, but significantly suppressed post-seasonal increases in nasal eosinophilia in subjects allergic to ragweed [329]. No serious adverse events were observed, and the investigators have since reported a «second season» protective effect against ragweed-induced symptoms. Other human trials for both allergic rhinitis and asthma are currently ongoing.

3.2.7.4 Infectious Diseases

Although this field in CpG research is relatively recent, evidence is beginning to accumulate for the therapeutic and prophylactic potentials of CpG ODNs in infectious disease. Promising effects of immunostimulatory ODNs have been described for bacterial, parasitical and viral infection settings. A selection of important studies using CpG ODNs in infectious disease models is represented in table 10, and the relevant findings on this exciting topic are summarized below.

3.2.7.4.1 Bacterial and Parasitical Infections

The first successful experiments concerning therapeutical use of CpGs against infectious disease was published in 1998 by Zimmermann and colleagues [330]. They studied the infection of mice with the parasite *Leishmania major* as a model for a lethal Th2-driven disease. In a first step, they could demonstrate prophylactic potential of CpG ODNs. CpG administration before infection with *L. major* coverted the immmune response in mice to a Th1-dominated phenotype including cytokine shift and antibody isotype switch. These responses were then shown to be associated with resistance against *L. major*-induced acute infection and provide protection against secondary infection. In a second experiment, Zimmerman and colleagues indicated efficacy of CpG ODNs in a post-exposure treatment against the infectious pathogen. CpG ODNs were curative when given as late as 20 days after lethal *L. major* infection. In the same way, specific CpG ODNs for the activation of human and simian cells were effective in reducing the severity of lesions caused by *Leishmania* infection of macaque monkeys [331]. The latter observations represented promising potential of CpGs in the treatment of infections in human beings.

Similarly to the findings linked to the *L. major* model, CpG ODN treatment has been associated with resistance in mice to intracellular bacteria. Inoculation of a single dose of CpG ODNs before infection of mice with a lethal dose of *Francisella tularensis* or *Listeria monocytogenes* induced protection against disease [332]. In addition, repeated administration of CpG ODNs conferred long term protection against both bacterial species [333].

Successful use of CpG ODNs in an infectious disease setting initially seemed to be restricted to infections with intracellular pathogens. However, recent works have extended these findings, demonstrating efficient treatment of extracellular microorganisms. In this way, it was shown that cellulitis in a mature chicken *E. coli* model could be prevented, indicating an immunoprophylactic effect of CpG

ODNs in this context [334]. Moreover, the same group described significantly increased survival rates of neonatal chicken challenged with a virulent isolate of *E. coli* inducing septicaemia, when they were prophylactically treated with CpG ODNs either at the stage of embryonated eggs or 2 days after birth [335]. A similar study demonstrated reduction of organ invasion by *Salmonella enteritidis* (SE) in one-day-old chickens pretreated with CpG ODNs as well as significantly reduced mortality of chickens with acute peritoneal infection due to SE [336].

These successful experiments in mice and birds indicate that CpG ODNs can promote both innate and pathogen-specific adaptive immune responses conferring to survival of lethal bacterial and parasitical challenges. The precise immunological requirements for CpG-induced protection of infection were slightly different in the models tested. However, a common feature described in all studies was the important antimicrobial function of IFN-γ and NK cells. By slowing the early growth and spread of pathogens, these CpG-induced features seem to improve the host's ability to mount a subsequent adaptive immune response, which provides effective protection against various bacterial and parasitical diseases.

3.2.7.4.2 Viral Infections

As viruses are intracellular pathogens, the resolution of most viral infections is associated with Th1 type immune responses characterized by CTL activity and production of IFN-γ. Since CpG ODNs are known to promote such responses, it appeared feasible to analyze their efficacy in viral infections.

Pyles and co-workers published in 2002 the first paper on a successful CpG ODN therapy against a viral infection [337]. They evaluated the effect of local CpG administration in a mouse and guinea pig model of vaginal *Herpes Simplex* virus type 2 (HSV-2) infection. A vaginal epithelial application of CpG ODNs, both before or shortly after infection, delayed disease onset and increased survival rates in mice challenged with a lethal dose of HSV-2. Furthermore, in the guinea pig model, an established infection could be successfully treated. Administration of CpG ODNs 21 days after HSV-2 infection reduced the frequency and severity of virus-induced lesions as well as the magnitude of viral shedding compared with control animals. Similarly, application of CpG ODNs was protective against *Influenza* virus [338]. Although mice exhibiting impaired Th1 type immune responses are highly susceptible to *Influenza* virus, treatment of such mice with CpG ODNs enabled the animals to rapidly clear virus from their lungs.

CpG ODNs have also been evaluated for their therapeutic potential against retroviral infections. The *Friend* leukaemia virus (FV) infection of mice is a powerful model to study general aspects of retroviral immunity. FV is a retroviral complex that can induce general immunosuppression and lethal erythroleukemia in mice. As with many other viral infections, resistance to FV-induced leukaemia in mice was associated with Th1-type immune responses. Enhancement of these responses during acute infection by a post-exposure treatment with CpG ODNs beginning 4 days after FV challenge infection led to prevention of 74% of the mice from developing acute leukaemia. CpG-mediated protection was associated with a significant reduction of viral loads in treated mice compared to those of control animals [339]. However, in stark contrast to the success of post-exposure treatment, CpG administration to mice before FV infection accelerated the development of virus-induced erythroleukemia. Furthermore, 70% of the animals from a mouse strain that was resistant to FV-induced leukaemia developed disease after inoculation with CpG ODNs before infection [340]. The explanation for these observations probably resides in the stimulation by CpG ODNs of the main target cell populations of FV, thus providing an enlarged target cell population for viral infection.

Since HIV in humans induces a Th2 cytokine dominance, it was hypothesized that treatment of HIV-1-infected patients with CpG ODNs may be a way to abolish the virus infection. Several *in vitro* experiments have been carried out to assess the therapeutic potential of CpGs in an HIV infection setting. Interestingly, the time point of CpG treatment of cells greatly influenced the outcome of experiments.

Literature

Pathogen	Animal Model	CpG ODN Type	Time Point of First Treatment
Parasite			
Leishmania major	Mouse	K	Before or at challenge
	Mouse	K	20 days post challenge
	Monkey	D	Before challenge
Plasmodium yoelli	Mouse	K and D	Before challenge
Bacteria			
Klebsiella	Mouse	K	24 hours before challenge
Mycobacterium Tuberculosis	Mouse	K	Before or at challenge
	Mouse	K	2 weeks post challenge
Listeria monocytogenes	Mouse	K	Before challenge
Franscisella tularensis	Mouse	K	Before challenge
Escherichia coli	Chicken	C	Before challenge
Salmonella enteritidis	Chicken	C	Before challenge
Virus			
Vaccinia Virus	Mouse	K and D	Before challenge
Human Papilloma Virus	Mouse	K	Post challenge
Herpes Simplex Virus Type 2	Mouse	K	Before or at challenge
	Guinea Pig	K	21 days post challenge
Friend Retrovirus	Mouse	K	4 days post challenge
	Mouse	K	Before challenge
Influenza Virus	Mouse	K	Before challenge
Reovirus Type 2	Mouse	K	Post challenge
Fungi			
Candida albicans	Mouse	D	3 days before challenge

Table 11: Application of CpG ODN in the context of various infectious diseases

Outcome	Reference
Protection against disease	330
Protection against disease	330
Protection against disease	331
Sterile Immunity	343
Improved survival	344
Attenuation of disease	345
Improved survival	
Protection against disease	332, 333
Protection against disease	332, 333
Improved survival	334, 335
Improved survival	336
Protection against disease	346
Reduction of tumor growth	347
Delayed disease onset	337
Attenuation of disease	337
Recovery of disease	339
Acceleration of disease	340
Protection against disease	338
Acceleration of autoimmune disease	348
Acceleration of disease	349

Literature

Schlaepfer and colleagues demonstrated that CpG ODNs, administered 2 days before or immediately upon infection, inhibited HIV replication nearly completely in lymphocyte cultures and prevented loss of CD4+ T cells [341]. Disappointingly though, control ODNs without CpG motifs also showed anti-HIV potential, indicating that the observed effects were non-specific and not due to TLR9 triggering. In another experiment, treatment of a latently infected T cell line with CpG ODNs stimulated expression of the pro-inflammatory cytokine NFκB and reactivated HIV replication, whereas no effects were evident when ODNs without CpG motifs were used. CpG-induced virus reactivation was blocked by chloroquine, indicating involvement of TLR9 in these observations [342]. Altogether, the non-specific anti-HIV activity of CpG ODNs, their ability to stimulate HIV replication in latently infected cells potentially leading to their subsequent elimination, as well as their documented ability to link innate and adaptive immune responses make them attractive candidates for further study as anti-HIV drugs.

In conclusion, CpG ODN treatment of viral infections seems dangerously double-sided in that it could result in an effective therapy but also in an acceleration of disease progression, depending on the time point of the treatment. Particular attention has to be attributed to treatment against viruses infecting haematopoetic cells activated by CpG ODNs, such as HIV, human T cell leukaemia, *Measles* virus, *Hepatitis B* and *Hepatitis C* viruses. Thus, the mechanisms of action of CpG ODNs must imperatively be precisely analyzed in animal models for such viral infections to test for negative side effects before designing clinical studies. An important step in this direction is the development of more defined immunostimulatory ODN molecules that stimulate only selected cell types of the immune system.

3.2.7.5 Use of CpG ODN as Vaccine Adjuvants

Vaccination remains to date the most effective method to prevent infectious diseases. CpG DNA improves the functional activity of professional APCs and triggers the production of cytokines and chemokines that support the development of adaptive immune responses. These considerations led many scientists to examine whether CpG ODNs could boost the immune response elicited by vaccines, promoting the immunogenicity of co-administered antigens.

Early experiments showed that adding CpG ODNs to conventional protein antigens, such as OVA, boosted both humoral and cell-mediated responses [350]. In these studies however, both OVA and ODNs could freely diffuse from the site of injection. The adjuvant properties of CpG ODNs were markedly improved in subsequent experiments when proximity of the ODNs to the antigen was maintained. Physically binding ODNs to antigen, linking the two with alum, or incorporating them into lipid emulsions or vesicles generated specific immune responses 10 to 1000-fold greater than with antigen alone [351, 352]. The increased adjuvant effects observed were attributed by the authors to a more efficient CpG-independent uptake, probably mediated by DNA-binding receptors on APCs.

Additional studies established that CpG ODNs could boost the response elicited by conventional vaccines. This effect is of particular relevance for pathogens in which a strong Th1 response is needed. When CpG ODNs were co-administered with vaccines against *Influenza* virus [353], *measles* virus [354], *Lymphocytic Choriomeningits* virus [355], *Hepatitis B* surface antigen [356], or *Tetanus* toxoid [357], preferential production of IFN-γ dependent IgG2a antibodies as well as development of antigen-specific CTL were observed. However, increased magnitude of vaccine-induced immune activity was not always associated with improved vaccine efficacy. In this way, mice treated with CpG ODNs plus a *Respiratory Syncytial* virus vaccine, for example, were only modestly protected from virus challenge and were at increased risk for pulmonary pathology [358].

Vaccine development was revolutionized by the finding that antigen-encoding DNA plasmids could induce cellular and humoral immune responses against foreign antigens. DNA vaccines are constructed with an antigen-encoding gene incorporated into a plasmid backbone of bacterial DNA. As plasmid vectors typically contain large numbers of immunostimulatory CpG motifs, it seemed relevant to examine their contribution to the observed immunological effects linked to DNA vaccination, such as production of large amounts of IFN-γ and IL-12. Treating plasmids with DNAse or Sss I methylase (selectively methylates the cytosine of CpG dinucleotides) uniformly eliminated cytokine production, indicating that the DNA is responsible for the cytokine release during such vaccination methods [359]. Additionally, the isotype of antigen-specific antibodies induced by plasmid vaccination was also examined after DNA vaccination, in order to assess possible effects of CpG motifs embedded in the plasmid. Mice immunized with a *Malaria* protein (CSP) emulsified in complete Freund's adjuvant primarily produce IgG1 anti-CSP antibodies. In contrast, injection of CSP-encoding DNA vaccines preferentially stimulated IgG2a antibody production [359]. As IFN-γ promotes IgM to IgG2a isotype switching, these findings are consistent with CpG-motif-induced IFN-γ production contributing to preferential production of IgG2a in immunized animals.

Subsequent studies demonstrated that both co-administration of CpG ODNs with DNA vaccines as well as engineering of additional CpG motifs into plasmid vectors significantly improved vaccine immunogenicity. Although adding CpG motifs to DNA vaccines appears to decrease the amount of vaccine required to induce antigen-specific antibody production, it seems that high numbers of CpG motifs are not always optimal. In this way, the immune response induced by a CpG-optimized plasmid is no greater than that of a conventional plasmid when both are administered at high concentrations [360]. Similarly, dose-response studies indicate that the ability of CpG ODNs to stimulate spleen cells to secrete cytokines and Ig *in vitro* reaches a plateau, and then begins to fall. In one report, introducing 16 additional CpG motifs into a DNA vaccine improved the humoral response elicited *in vivo*, while introducing 50 such motifs reduced the response [361]. These findings suggest that the maximal effect of CpG motifs may require relatively low doses of DNA. Moreover, the adjuvant effect is greatest when antigen dose is limited. Indeed, modest adjuvanticity was observed when large amounts of antigen was delivered [362]. This phenomenon is referred to as the antigen-sparing effect of CpG DNA.

Two main clinical trials in which CpG ODNs were used as vaccine adjuvants have been described. The first was a double blind study in which CpG ODNs were co-administered many times with Energix B, the licensed *Hepatitis B* vaccine. Healthy adult volunteers immunized with the vaccine plus CpG ODNs developed significantly higher mean antibody titres, more rapidly than those immunized with vaccine alone. In the second double blind study, CpG ODNs were co-administered with Fluarix *Influenza* virus vaccine. Inclusion of CpG ODNs did not increase antibody response of naïve recipients when compared to Fluarix alone, but increased antibody titres among individuals with pre-existing *Influenza* virus-specific antibodies. Moreover, PBMCs from CpG ODN-vaccinated subjects responded to *in vitro* re-stimulation by secreting markedly higher levels of IFN-γ than the PBMCs from control vaccines.

Altogether, these observations indicate a vast potential for use of CpG as adjuvants in immunization studies for a wide variety of diseases in different species. Future studies will allow determination of optimal structure and dose of CpG ODN in combination with vaccines, thus enhancing efficacy of currently used protocols or initiating new possibilities in areas where vaccination methods have to date not been successful.

3.2.7.6 Safety Concerns

Several potential safety issues are raised by the use of CpG ODNs as immunoprotective agents. Concerns regarding enhancement of the immunogenicity of self proteins at the site of delivery, thereby triggering the development of autoimmune disease, as well as production of cytokines that may increase host susceptibility to other harmful agents, have mainly attracted attention during trials on mice.

The ability of CpG DNA to promote the development of autoimmune disease is supported by studies showing that bacterial DNA can elicit the production of anti-double-stranded DNA auto-antibodies in normal mice [363] and accelerate the development of immune disease in lupus-prone animals [364]. CpG DNA also stimulates the production of IL-6 and blocks the apoptotic death of activated lymphocytes. Both these functions are known to predispose to the development of autoimmune disease by facilitating the persistence of self-reactive lymphocytes.

There is also evidence that CpG ODNs enhance the production of TNF-α, a cytokine associated with the development of life-threatening toxic shock. When CpG ODNs were administered together with other agents that promote TNF-α release (such as LPS or D-galactosamine), severe mortality and morbidity were observed [365].

A more recent report showed that daily administration of CpG ODNs for three weeks can cause dramatic changes in the architecture of the primary lymph organs and induce haemorrhagic ascites and multifocal liver necrosis [294]. However, given the relatively long duration CpG ODN-induced immunological effects (days to weeks), daily treatment over long periods of time should not be required. Earlier studies had examined whether toxicity might occur under more normal circumstances: CpG ODNs at doses equal to or exceeding that typically used in adjuvant experiments was injected weekly for 4 months into normal mice. No adverse health effects were observed in any of the animals and none showed macroscopic or microscopic evidence of tissue damage or inflammation [360]. Similarly, no undesired effects were noted in studies involving delivery of CpG ODNs to non-human primates [366]. Thus, although concern remains that CpG ODNs might have adverse effects under certain conditions, there is to date no evidence that CpG ODN administration is toxic to normal, healthy animals, when following a protocol designed to provide protection from infection.

CpG ODNs have been considered safe enough and are authorized for clinical trials in animals as well as in humans. Clinical studies are proceeding with subjects being closely monitored for the development of adverse reactions. To date, toxicity has not been observed in normal animals or humans when CpG ODNs were used as immunoprotective agents, vaccine adjuvants, or therapeutic instruments, suggesting a promising future for more common use of CpGs in various disease settings.

4. Material and Methods

4.1 Objectives

The following experiments and objectives were pursued in the course of this study:

- Prophylactic treatment over a period of 5 consecutive days of spf cats using either dSLIM™, an optimally synthesized molecule containing various CpG motifs, or a placebo substance

- Challenge infection of all cats with the FIV-Glasgow 8 (GL8) strain

- Characterization of the host's immune response both during treatment and after challenge infection, by assessment of relevant cytokine responses in whole blood, as well as evaluation of the potential to produce various cytokines by PBMCs isolated from whole blood of the cats and stimulated *in vitro*

- Determination of the degree of protection elicited by the treatment, through analysis of various immunological and virological parameters in the cats such as seroconversion, infectious virus isolation, proviral and viral load mesurments in peripheral blood lymphocytes and plasma

- Evaluation of treatment effect on the transmission potential of FIV infection, by examination of excreted viral loads in saliva

Material and Methods

4.2 General Information and Important Methods

Several methods have been repeatedly used in the laboratory during the course of the experiment. Brief theoretical indications, including aim and principals of these methods, as well as material used, are described below.

4.2.1 Enzyme-Linked Immunosorbent Assay

ELISA is a sensitive immunoassay which uses an enzyme linked to an antibody or antigen as a marker for the detection of a specific protein, often another antigen or antibody. It is often used as a diagnostic test to determine exposure to a particular infectious agent, by identifying antibodies or antigen present in a blood sample. In the case of FIV, antibodies against the TM or the SU glycoproteins are commonly detected, and have proven to give sensitive indications to the presence of an infection in cats [152]. For this purpose, recombinant FIV SU or TM proteins are mixed with a coating buffer and allowed to bind to the bottom of microtitre plate wells. The plates are incubated for 3 hours at 37°C and then overnight at 4°C, to allow complete binding of the antigens. They are subsequently washed with a special ELISA wash buffer containing NaCl and Tween-20 (polyoxyethylene sorbitan monolaurate), filled with PBS, and stored at -20 °C until use.

Feline plasma samples are added to the wells and allowed to complex with the bound antigen. Unbound products are then removed with several washes of PBS. Goat anti-cat antibodies labeled with HRP, are allowed to bind to the captured antibodies from the cat plasma samples, and unbound products are again washed out several times with ELISA wash buffer. The assay is then quantified by measuring the amount of labeled antibody bound to the matrix through the use of ABTS (2,2'-azo-bis(3-ethylbenzthiazoline-6-sulfonic acid), a colorimetric substrate of HRP. Optical density (OD) of each sample is then determined by an absorbance reader, and the results are compared to positive controls in order to confirm or reject presence of antibodies to FIV. A major advantage of this technique is that the plasma samples measured must not be specifically treated prior to use. Moreover, these assays are very sensitive, rendering them reliable for diagnostic and research purposes. Complementary information about use of ELISA in this experiment can be found under 4.4.4.2.1.

4.2.2 Nucleic Acid Extractions

Extraction of nucleic acids from the collected samples is necessary for subsequent specific quantitative analysis by PCR. For this purpose, the nucleic acid extraction apparatus MagNa Pure[1] was used in this study, and corresponding protocols, recommended by the manufacturer, were followed. The isolation and purification of total nucleic acids (TNA), as well as mRNA were accomplished on several occasions during the course of this experiment. Both procedures are based on magnetic bead particles (MGP) technology.

During TNA extraction, DNA as well as RNA are isolated. In a first step, addition of lysis/binding buffer to the sample results in a complete lysis of proteins by denaturation. DNA and RNA are released and simultaneously stabilized. Proteinase K is then added to the sample and starts digestion of the denatured proteins. Next, TNA molecules bind to the surface of added MGPs, due to the high ionic strength of the previously attached lysis/binding buffer. Several washes with specific wash buffers remove impurities like denatured proteins and cellular debris from the sample to finally allow elution of purified TNA.

Extraction of mRNA relies on the presence of a poly-adenosine (A) tail at the 3' end of mRNA molecules. A first lysis step allows release of mRNA and inactivation of nucleases present in the sample. The lysate is incubated with a capture buffer, which consists of biotin-labelled oligo dT diluted in a specific hybridization substance. The latter allows the biotin-labelled oligo dT to bind to the poly-A residues of mRNA. The complexes thus formed are then immobilized onto the surfaces of streptavidin-coated magnetic beads (SMP). Unbound substances are removed by several washing steps

---

1. Roche Diahnostics, Rotkreuz, Switzerland

Material and Methods

and addition of DNase solution allows to digest DNA present in the sample. Finally, the purified mRNA is eluted.

4.2.3 Real-Time Fluorogenic Polymerase Chain Reaction

The conventional PCR allows exponential increase in the amount of copies of a desired gene in a determined number of amplification cycles. Flanking regions of the desired sequence must be known in order to design oligonucleotide primers which can hibridize to the beginning and the end of the target. A thermophilic enzyme, the Taq DNA polymerase, purified from the hot springs bacterium *Thermus aquaticus*, then catalyzes specific DNA synthesis directed from the primers. Amplification cycles consist each in temperature variations allowing three fundamental steps:

- Denaturation of the DNA strand: the solution is heated at 95°C for 15 seconds

- Hybridization or annealing of two primers (one is a reverse primer and the other is a forward primer): the solution is quickly cooled to 54°C to let the primers anneal to a DNA strand; one primer anneals to the 3' end of the target while the other primer anneals to the 3' end of the complementary target strand

- DNA synthesis or elongation: the solution is then heated to 72°C, the optimal temperature for Taq DNA polymerase

All 3 steps above are considered as one cycle; amplification of a DNA template is usually done over 45 cycles. A thermal cycler programmed with a protocol that goes through all three steps of a cycle for the desired amount of cycles is used for PCR reactions in general.

In order to amplify a RNA sequence, complementary DNA (cDNA) has to be

Material and Methods

synthesized using a RT enzyme before initiation of the standard PCR described above. Incubation for 1 hour at 37ºC, the optimal temperature for the RT, is needed for this additional step.

The real-time PCR is a more recent system allowing not only amplification, but also quantification of a DNA or RNA sequence using a fluorescent reporter [367]. In addition to a forward and a reverse primer, an oligonucleotide, called probe, which specifically binds to the target sequence between the hybridization sites of the primers, must be added to the reaction. Importantly, a reporter fluorescent dye and a quencher dye are attached to the probe. While the probe is intact, the spacial proximity of the quencher greatly reduces the fluorescence emitted by the reporter dye. During amplification however, annealing of the probe to its target sequence generates a substrate that is cleaved by the 5' nuclease activity of Taq DNA polymerase when the enzyme extends from an upstream primer into the region of the probe. This cleavage of the probe separates the reporter dye from the quencher dye, increasing the reporter dye signal. Simultaneously, the probe is removed from the target strand, allowing primer extension to continue to the end of the template strand. Additional reporter dye molecules are cleaved from their respective probes with each cycle, inducing a logarithmic increase in fluorescence intensity proportional to the amount of template produced. Principles of the real-time PCR are shown in figure 9.

The ABI PRISM 7700 Sequence Detection System[2] is a flexible system designed to take full advantage of the benefits of fluorogenic probe detection. The 7700 system has a built-in thermal cycler and a laser directed via fiber optic cables to each of 96 sample wells. The fluorescence emission travels back through the cables to a camera detector. At the end of a determined amount of cycles, data is stored and fluorescence intensity of each sample can be visualized.

---

2. Applied Biosystems, Foster City, CA, USA

Material and Methods

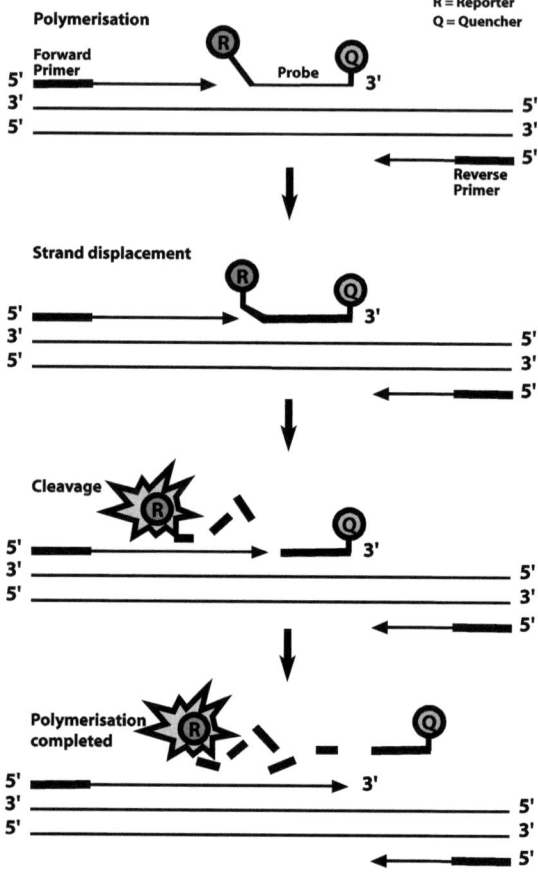

Figure 9: The principles of Real-Time PCR

4.2.3.4 Peripheral Blood Mononuclear Cell Isolation

For *in vitro* analyses concerning FIV, it is essential to isolate and cultivate successfully PBMCs, as they are the targets of infection. For this purpose, the Ficoll-Hypaque gradient separation of cells from whole blood is commonly used [361]. Due to the density gradient, centrifugation of whole blood carefully layered on Ficoll-Hypaque, allows separation of different blood components as shown in figure 10.

Material and Methods

In our experiment, PBMC isolation was accomplished using the following protocol:

- Feline ethylenediaminetetraacaetic acid (EDTA)-treated blood was collected in evacuated tubes and centrifuged for 10 minutes at 1500rpm. Plasma was aspirated and replaced by the same volume of HBSS 1x

- Hank's balanced salt solution (HBSS) was carefully mixed with the blood and the mixture was slowly poured over 4 ml Histopaque®[3] previously displaced in a 15ml conical centrifuge tube

- A gradient was created by centrifugation at 2000rpm for 25 minutes

- The buffy coat fraction was collected and washed in 10ml HBSS previously aliquoted in 15ml centrifuge tubes

- The cells were pelleted by centrifugation at 1200rpm for 10 minutes

- Complete Roswell Park Memorial Institute (RPMI) medium (RPMI 1640 supplemented with 10 % feotal calf serum (FCS), Glutamin, 1U Penicillin, 100µg/ml Streptomycin, 2,7% Sodium Bicarbonate) was used for resuspension and further cultivation of the cells

- 10µg conA[4]/ml of cell culture were added to promote IL-2 receptor expression on the surface of the cells

- After 24 hours incubation of the cells at 37°C, 5% CO_2, 20U

---

3. Sigma, St.Louis, MO, USA
4. Sigma, St.Louis, MO, USA

Material and Methods

IL-2 / ml culture was added in order to stimulate proliferation and survival of the cells

- Medium was partially replaced by fresh IL-2-supplemented complete RPMI every 3 days

PBMCs treated in this way generally survive a total of 4 to 6 weeks.

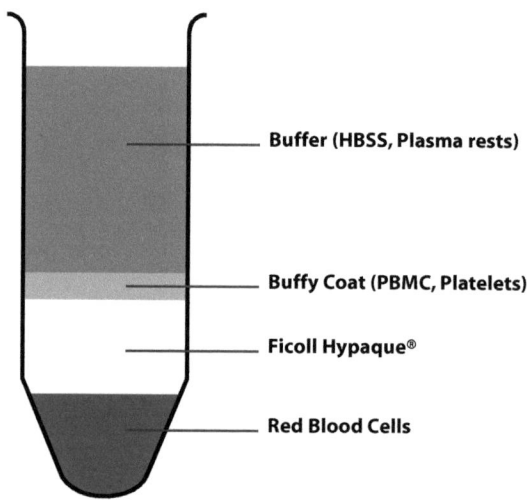

Figure 10: PBMC isolation by Ficoll-Hypaque® gradient

4.3 Pre-experiment Formalities

4.3.1 Cats

A total of 20 male spf domestic cats were shipped from Liberty Research Inc.[5] at approximately 10 weeks of age. They were divided at their arrival into 2 groups of 10 cats each, equally distributing individuals according to their age and litter

---

5. Waverly, NY, USA

provenance. Thus, the average age of the cats in both groups was 9.9 weeks. Each group was housed separately, in an animal-friendly environment and under optimal ethological conditions.

4.3.2 Adaptation Period and Assessment of Health Status

An adaptation period of 8 weeks permitted the establishment of essential social trust between the cats and the persons responsible for the experiment. With the intention of ensuring minimal levels of stress for the animals, great importance was attributed to daily visiting and playing with the cats during this period as well as during the entire duration of the experiment.

In order to certify their health status was in conformity with the standards of the experiment, the cats were clinically examined by a veterinarian shortly after their arrival. At the same time, EDTA-supplemented and heparin-supplemented blood samples were collected under light anaesthesia (see 4.4.3) to rule out possible haematological and biochemical deviations, as well as direct presence of FeLV or FIV infections. Serum samples were also tested for presence of antibodies to feline parvovirus (FPV), feline coronavirus (FCoV), feline herpesvirus (FHV), and feline calicivirus (FCV) and FIV as well as presence of p27, a marker protein for FeLV viremia. Additionally, oropharyngeal, ocular and rectal swabs were collected, in order to test for undesired occurrence of FPV, FCoV, FHV, FCV.

Haematological status was assessed from EDTA-supplemented blood using the Cell Dyn 3500 (CD 3500) Haematology Analyser[6] and clinical chemistry parameters were tested in heparinated plasma by the Cobas Integra 800 Analyzer[7] after centrifugation of the blood samples at 3000rpm for 10 minutes. For the testing of presence of retroviral infections (FIV and FeLV), TNA was extracted

---

5. Waverly, NY, USA
6. Abbott Diagnostics, Santa Clara, CA, U
7. Roche Diagnostics, Rotkreuz, Switzerland

Material and Methods

from EDTA- supplemented whole blood samples according to the manufacturer's recommendation[8], and real-time PCR analyses[9] were subsequently carried out under conditions described elsewhere [369, 370].

Cotton swabs with plastic stems were either applied to the medial corner of both eyes for the collection of ocular secretions, rubbed against the gums and inner cheek pouches in the mouth or introduced into the rectum for collection of oropharyngeal and rectal material respectively. Persons responsible for collecting these samples held only the plastic stems and carefully avoided touching the cotton swab, in order to minimize contamination. At the time of collection, the swabs were immediately placed in 1,5ml Eppendorf tubes, with the cotton swab thereby facing the bottom of the tube. In order to prepare the samples for subsequent TNA extraction, 200µl of HBSS were first added to each Eppendorf tube, before incubation at 42°C for 10 minutes to moisten the swabs. After centrifugation at 8000rpm for 1 minute, the swabs were inversed in the tubes so that the cotton part was facing upward, and centrifuged again for 1 minute at 8000rpm, to ensure that an optimal amount of material was now contained in the HBSS. The swabs were then discarded and 300µl of TNA lysis buffer were added to each sample before proceeding to TNA extraction according to the manufacturer's recommendations[10]. Extracted material from rectal swabs was analyzed for the presence of FPV and FCoV, and extracted material from ocular and oropharyngeal swabs was tested for presence of FCV and FHV using real-time PCR[11]. The assays and PCR conditions used for these measurements have been published in the past 10 years [371-373].

4.4 Course of the study

The total duration of the present experiment was of 12 weeks. Treatment protocols, challenge method, as well as description of subsequent sample collections and

---

8. MagNA Pure LC TNA isolation kit, Roche GmbH, Mannheim, Germany
9. ABI Prism 7700 sequence detector, Applied Biosystems, Foster City, CA, USA
10. MagNA Pure LC TNA isolation kit, Roche GmbH, Mannheim Germany
11. ABI Prism 7700 sequence detector, Applied Biosystems, Foster City, CA, USA

Material and Methods

laboratory work are detailed below. Time points of these different steps are represented in figure 11.

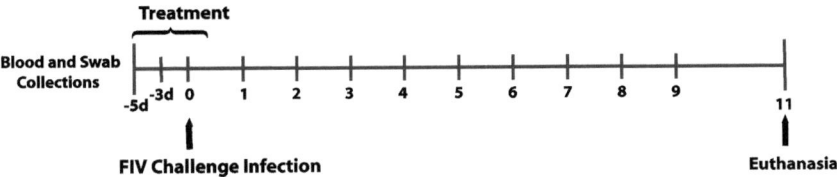

Figure 11: Schedule of the study

4.4.1 Treatment Protocol

For the prophylactic treatment of the cats against subsequent FIV challenge, dSLIM™ was provided by Mologen AG[12]. dSLIM™ is a non-coding DNA sequence of immunomodulating conformation comprising non-methylated CpG dinucleotide motifs. Figure 12 shows the configuration of this covalently-closed dumbbell-shaped double stem-loop molecule. The ODN of dSLIM™ are linked with a phosphodiester backbone, and its particular dumbbell-shaped structure allows protection of the open ends of the ODN against degradation by DNases. This additionally permits to avoid the use of phosphorothioate as backbone modification, which is linked to a series of unfavourable side effects (see 3.2.6).

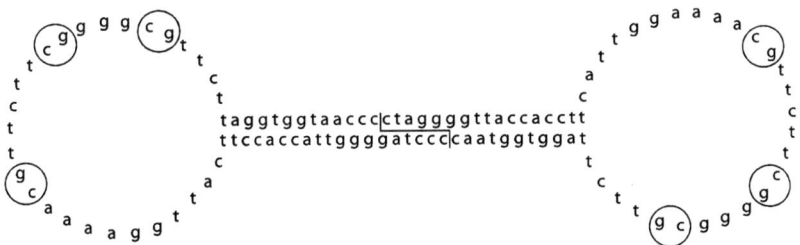

Figure 12: Schematic representation of the dSLIM™ molecule

12. Berlin, Germany

Material and Methods

In vitro and *in vivo* experiments with dSLIM™ have indicated that this molecule possesses the biological and immunological properties of a typical C-type CpG ODN described in section 3.2.6. Importantly, successful immunomodulation of both murine and human cells have demonstrated that the effect of dSLIM ™ is not restricted to one species. Furthermore, repeated injection of dSLIM™ into mice induced no adverse reactions or signs of toxicity, and several human clinical trials confirmed the safety of its administration *in vivo* [374].

In this study, 10 cats were treated with dSLIM™ on 5 consecutive days before challenge infection, using the following protocol.

Day of treatment	Mode of Administration	dSLIM™ Concentration	Volume
1	s.c	1mg/ml	0.75ml
2	s.c	1mg/ml	0.75ml
3	s.c	1mg/ml	0.75ml
4	i.v and s.c	0.1* and 1mg/ml**	1.5* and 0.75ml**
5	i.p	0.1mg/ml	3ml

Table 12: Administration protocol of dSLIM™ *in vivo* for the 5-day treatment period prior to FIV challenge infection. s.c: subcutaneous, i.v: intravenous, i.p:intraperitoneal (*i.v, **s.c)

The 10 remaining cats were treated simultaneously with subcutaneous injections of a placebo (phosphate-buffered saline, PBS).

4.4.2 Challenge Infection

The challenge infection was carried out 24 hours after the last treatment injection. After rapid thawing of the viral stock and preparation of individual doses on ice, all cats were infected intraperitoneally with 50 cat infectious doses 50 (50 CID_{50}) of the GL8 strain of FIV previously titrated *in vivo*[13].

---

13. kindly provided by Dr. Magaret Hosie and Prof. O. Jarret, University of Glasgow, Great Britain

4.4.3 Clinical Examinations, Blood and Oropharyngeal Swab collections

The cats were thoroughly clinically examined by a veterinarian and blood samples were collected just before the first treatment injection in order to obtain base values of the parameters subsequently analyzed in the course of the experiment. Auscultations were carried out daily during the treatment period and additional blood samples were collected on the third day of treatment, allowing assessment of any clinical symptoms or haematological and immune alterations initiated by the injections of dSLIM™. On the morning before challenge infection, the cats were again clinically examined, and one oropharyngeal swab per cat was collected in addition to the blood samples. From this time point on, clinical examinations, as well as blood and oropharyngeal swab collections were performed weekly for a total of 11 weeks, with the exception of the 10th week. 2 ml each of heparin and EDTA-supplemented blood were thereby collected, as certain subsequent analyses imperatively required either one of these anti-coagulants.

In order to minimize the stress conferred to the cats during the sample collections, they were administered a combination of 0,2 ml/kg ketamin[14] and 0,02 ml/kg midazolam[15], inducing short term anaesthesia. The doses were adapted to the weights of the growing cats throughout the experiment. Apart from gradual resistance to ketamin leading to slightly reduced anaesthetical efficacy over time, no undesired side effects linked to this combination were observed.

4.4.4 Laboratory Analysis of Relevant Host and Viral Parameters

4.4.4.1 Haematology and Clinical Chemistry

On the same day as each blood collection, the blood cell count of each cat was measured from 400μl of EDTA-supplemented blood using the CD 3500 Haematology Analyser[16]. Clinical chemistry parameters were analyzed by the Cobas

---

14. Narketan®10, Vetoquinol AG, Belp, CH
15. Dormicum®, Roche Pharma AG, Reinach, CH
16. Abbott Diagnostics, Santa Clara, CA, USA

Material and Methods

Integra system[17] using 500µl heparinated plasma obtained after centrifugation of the blood samples at 3000rpm for 10 minutes.

4.4.4.2 Evaluation of Host Immune Parameters

In this study, the induction of immune responses was mainly assessed by the determination of seroconversion after challenge infection and by the quantitative and comparative analyses of cytokine levels produced during both the treatment period and after FIV challenge.

4.4.4.2.1 Seroconversion

Antibodies directed against the FIV TM protein were measured with ELISA under conditions described elsewhere [152]. Briefly, recombinant FIV TM antigens[18] were pre-coated on ELISA plates, and goat anti-cat IgG conjugated to HRP[19] was used as conjugate. Presence of anti-TM antibodies in 15µl feline plasma samples was determined by absorbance measured in a Spectra max PLUS ELISA reader[20]. To standardize OD values between different runs, standard positive and negative control sera respectively collected from an experimentally FIV-ZH2-infected cat with high antibody titres, and from a non-infected spf cat were included in every run. All samples were tested in duplicates, and OD values of plasma samples from our cats were expressed as percentage of the positive control OD value. General information about this method can be viewed under 4.2.1.

4.4.4.2.2 Determination of Cytokine Expression

The expression of both IL-12 and IL-10 were tested as indicators for Th1 and

---

17. Roche Diagnostics, Rotkreuz, Switzerland
18. previously produced in our laboratory by Dr. J. Huder
19. Jackson Immunoresearch Laboratories, Bar Harbour, Main, USA
20. Biotech AG, Basel

Material and Methods

Th2 immune responses respectively, and quantification of glyceraldehyde-3-phosphatedehydrogenase (GAPDH), a catalytic enzyme produced by a so-called «housekeeping» gene, allowed standardization of these measurements. An inherent assumption in the use of housekeeping genes is that expression of these genes remains constant in the cells or tissues under investigation. Apart from its important role in gylcolysis, GAPDH was reported to be involved in the processes of DNA replication, DNA repair, nuclear RNA export, membrane fusion and microtubule bundling. Most importantly, GAPDH is known to be ubiquitously expressed in stable quantities within a healthy individual. Although its production rate may diverge between tissues or cells analyzed and in the course of different pathologies, age and gender have been shown not to alter this gene's expression.

With the objective to investigate whether treatment and/or infection resulted in altered production or «production potential» of these cytokines, their mRNA levels in PBMCs were measured in 2 separate experiments described below. It must additionally be noted here that presence of IL-12 in our study was determined by detection of mRNA for the p40 subunit of this cytokine. The PCR assays and conditions used in this study have been developed previously in our laboratory [375, 376].

4.4.4.2.2.1 Cytokine Measurements in Whole Blood

Immediately after collecting the blood from each cat, 100µl EDTA-supplemented blood was mixed with 300µl of previously aliquoted mRNA lysis buffer. The samples were stored at -80°C until further analysis.

mRNA was extracted according to the manufacturer's recommendations[21]. Finally, real-time PCR analysis[22] of GAPDH, IL-12 and IL-10 in the extracted samples was performed simultaneously with previously prepared standard dilutions of each cytokine, in order to assure quantitative measurements.

---

21. MagNA Pure LC mRNA isolation kit, Roche GmbH, Mannheim Germany
22. ABI Prism 7700 sequence detector, Applied Biosystems, Foster City, CA, USA

Material and Methods

4.4.4.2.2.2 Cytokine Measurements in Stimulated and Unstimulated PBMCs

The aim of this experiment was to determine whether PBMCs of treated cats revealed greater potential to produce specific cytokines *in vitro*, in comparison to PBMCs of control cats. It seemed relevant to further assess the influence of FIV infection on this potential.

In order to pursue this objective, PBMCs from each individual cat were isolated at 2 different time points during the experiment, namely on the day of FIV infection, and at week 8 post-challenge. The purified PBMCs were then distributed in 3 different wells of a 24-well plate, each well containing 5×10^5 cells in a total volume of 1 ml complete RPMI 1640 with Glutamax I[TM23] (equivalent to L-glutamin) supplemented with 20U recombinant IL-2/ml culture. The PBMCs in the three different wells were treated as follows:

1. Unstimulated: addition of 10µl complete RPMI 1640 with Glutamax™ I
2. Stimulated with ConA: addition of 10µg ConA[24]
3. Stimulated with LPS: addition of 1µg LPS[25]

ConA is a lectin protein from the jackbean (*Canavalia ensiformis*), and LPS is a major suprastructure of the membrane of Gram-negative bacteria. Both are known to be potent lymphocyte mitogens.

After 24 hours of incubation at 37°C and 5% CO_2, the cells were harvested by centrifugation of the plates at 2000rpm for 12 minutes, the supernatant was removed, and 400µl mRNA lysis buffer was added to the cells. Until further analysis, the lysed cells were then stored at -80°C in labelled 1,5ml Eppendorf tubes.

---

23. GIBCO®, Invitrogen, Carlsbad, CA, USA
24. Sigma, St.Louis, MO, USA
25. Sigma, St.Louis, MO, USA

mRNA was later on extracted[26], and quantitative analysis of GAPDH, IL-10 and IL-12 p40 was performed as described above (4.4.4.2.2.1).

4.4.4.3 Evolution of FIV Infection

The degree of protection of the cats against the challenge FIV infection was evaluated with indicators for host-virus contact, as well as for both established and productive infection. Early detectable host response to foreign antigen can be assessed by the presence and level of antibodies in plasma. Further transgression of the host's early immunity barriers is measured by integration of viral genome in target lymphocytes. Viremia and presence of virus in saliva indicate in turn effective viral replication and liberation of virions. Capacity of these newly produced viral particles to infect target cells is crucial to viral survival within the host and transmission to other cats. The analyses described below were thus designed to evaluate the effect of treatment on the evolution of FIV infection in the host.

4.4.4.3.1 Measurements of Proviral and Viral Loads in Blood

In order to determine the FIV proviral load in the cats' PBMCs in a comparable manner between individuals, TNA was extracted[27] from a whole blood volume containing 10^6 white blood cells (WBC), and subsequently analyzed by real-time PCR[28]. The total WBC count from the weekly haematological analysis permitted to estimate the volume needed for extraction. TNA extractions were carried out as recommended by the manufacturer, and the maximal blood volume thereby used was 200μl. In cases where 10^6 WBC were comprised in less than 200μl, HBSS was added to compensate for the missing volume.

The detection of the FIV load in plasma was determined with similar methods.

---

26. MagNA Pure LC mRNA isolation kit, Roche GmbH, Mannheim Germany
27. MagNA Pure LC TNA isolation kit, Roche GmbH, Mannheim, Germany
28. ABI Prism 7700 sequence detector, Applied Biosystems, Foster City, CA, USA

Material and Methods

TNA was first extracted[29] from plasma samples obtained by centrifugation of 500 µl EDTA- supplemented blood at 3500rpm, for 10 minutes. These samples, together with previously established standard dilutions, were then analyzed by quantitative real-time RT-PCR[30].

4.4.4.3.2 Isolation of Virus from Plasma

Presence of infectious virus in plasma from our infected cats was determined between weeks 2 and 8 of the study, with the exception of week 6. On each of these weeks, a PBMC culture with blood from 2 spf cats was established 2 days before blood collection. 24 hours after their isolation, the cells were stimulated with 20U IL-2/ml culture. On the day of blood collection, the cells were distributed into the wells of a 24-well plate, at a concentration of $5x10^5$ cells per well. 500µl of heparin-supplemented blood collected from our cats was centrifuged twice consecutively at 3000rpm for 10 minutes, in order to minimize cellular contamination of the samples. 100µl of obtained plasma was then added to one well for each individual cat. Plasma of the same spf cats from which the PBMCs were isolated served as negative control, and FIV-GL8 from our viral stock was used as positive control. After incubation of the inoculated cells at 37°C, 5 % CO_2 for 3 hours, 600µl of fresh, complete RPMI medium supplemented with 13 U IL-2 were added. The cells then remained in culture for 4 weeks. Once a week, 500µl was collected from the cultures and replaced by 500µl complete RPMI freshly supplemented with 10U IL-2. The samples obtained were centrifuged at 3000rpm for 10 minutes, and the supernatant was separated from the cell pellet before storage at -80°C. Later on, TNA was extracted[31] from the supernatant samples thus collected on the fourth week post-inoculation, according to the manufacturer's recommendation. The presence of FIV RNA was analyzed by real-time RT-PCR[32].

---

29. MagNA Pure LC TNA isolation kit, Roche GmbH, Mannheim, Germany
30. ABI Prism 7700 sequence detector, Applied Biosystems, Foster City, CA, USA
31. MagNA Pure LC TNA isolation kit, Roche GmbH, Mannheim, Germany
32. ABI Prism 7700 sequence detector, Applied Biosystems, Foster City, CA, USA

4.4.4.3.3 Measurements of Viral Load in Saliva

The oropharyngeal swabs collected weekly were prepared for TNA extraction as described above (4.3.2). TNA was extracted[33] according to the manufacturer's recommendations. The samples thus obtained were analyzed for presence of FIV RNA by real-time RT-PCR[34].

4.4.5 Statistical Analysis

All the results obtained in the course of the study were entered in Microsoft® Excel 2000 for further evaluation. Haematological and biochemical blood values, as well as host immune and viral parameters were subsequently analyzed using appropriate statistical programs[35].

---

33. MagNA Pure LC TNA isolation kit, Roche GmbH, Mannheim, Germany
34. ABI Prism 7700 sequence detector, Applied Biosystems, Foster City, CA, USA
35. Stat view for Windows, version 5.0, Graph Pad Prism®, version 3.0

5. Results

Regular clinical examinations of the cats and fluid laboratory work permitted the collection of a great amount of data during the course of this study. Clinical examinations and blood collections took place on a weekly basis and for a total of 11 weeks (with the exception of week 10), starting from the time point of FIV challenge infection (week 0, w0). Additional data were collected during the treatment, namely 3 days before challenge (week 0 -3 days, w0-3d), as well as immediately before the onset of the treatment, 5 days before challenge (week 0-5 days, w0-5d). In order to allow optimal comparison of clinical observations and experimental results obtained from both groups, the collected data were represented first graphically, and then thoroughly analyzed by the appropriate statistical tests.

The graphics displayed in this section show mean group values obtained for distinct parameters evaluated during the study. For clearer understanding, standard deviations are not shown in the graphics. However, particularly high variations within the groups, as well as exceptional individual cases are mentioned when necessary. Only those graphics either representing the parameters for which significant differences between groups were observed, or demonstrating other relevant elements, have been selected to illustrate this chapter.

All collected data were tested for normal distribution using the Kolmogorov-Smirnov test, and subsequently analyzed according to this test's results. In this way, data from both groups, showing normal distribution in every week, were then compared using a Student's T-test for each week separately. In contrast, data which failed to show normal distribution in one or more weeks were evaluated for each week separately, by the Mann Whitney U-test. Parametrical data collected for each

Results

group was also statistically evaluated for significance in alterations over time. All comparative results thus obtained were systematically considered significant when p>0.05. Significant differences between the groups are illustrated in the graphics by a star (✶). Also, selected significant alterations over time are indicated in the diagrams by a bracket (✶). All other significant parametrical alterations are described in the text only, in order to avoid confusion in the figures.

5.1 Clinical Examination

5.1.1 Body Weight

The cats were weighed during weekly blood collections. The effects of the conferred anaesthesia enabled to obtain more precise values. The mean weight values of both groups increased continuously during the entire duration of the study, as normally expected for young, growing cats. At the beginning of the experiment, weight differences between both groups were noted (figure 13). Indeed, during the treatment (w0-3d) and at the time point of the challenge infection (w0), the mean body weight of the dSLIM™-treated group was significantly lower than that of the control group. However, as of week 1 already, the mean body weight values of both groups followed very similar curves until the end of the study.

5.1.2 Body Temperature

The body temperature of each cat was measured weekly on the occasion of blood collections, immediately after the onset of the sedation effects. Although minimal fluctuations were observed, the differences between mean values of both groups showed no significance during the entire duration of the study (figure 14).

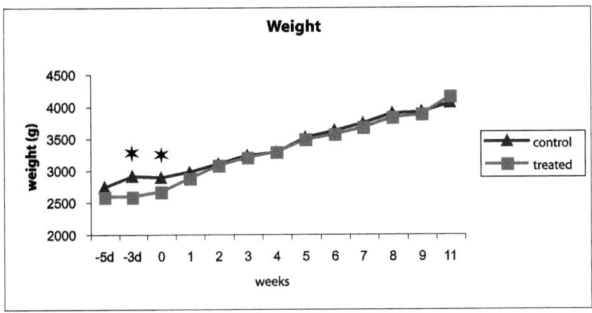

Figure 13: Mean body weights in grams (g)

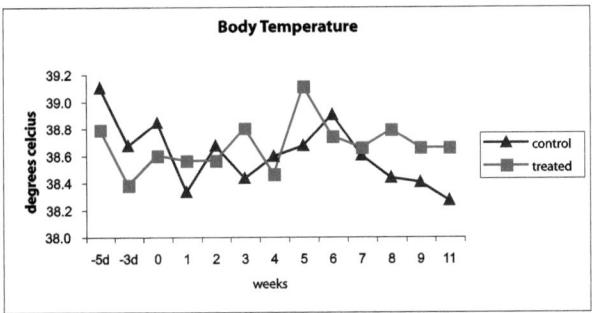

Figure 14: Mean body temperatures in degrees celcius (°C)

5.1.3 Clinical Symptoms

As dSLIM™ had never before been systemically administered to domestic cats, it appeared to be of great importance to closely examine the cats during the treatment period, in order to assess any reaction to the injections. Particular attention was given to general symptoms of discomfort, such as apathy or loss of appetite, as well as to systemic and local inflammatory reactions. Regardless of the method of administration of dSLIM™, the treated cats presented no local or systemic adverse reactions at any time during the 5 days of treatment, and no behavioral differences were observed when they were compared to the control group.

Results

As of the time point of FIV challenge, special attention was attributed, during weekly examinations, to possible delayed reactions to the treatment, and to typical signs of acute FIV infection. The first abnormal clinical symptoms appeared however no earlier than 3 weeks after the challenge infection. Most cats of both groups presented slightly enlarged mandibular lymph nodes. By week 5 after challenge infection, enlargement of the popliteal lymph nodes was also observed. These clinical signs persisted throughout the 11 weeks of the study, and no significant differences could be determined between both groups, neither in the number of cats presenting the symptoms, nor in the number of lymph nodes enlarged per cat. Moreover, during the necropsy, which took place 11 weeks after challenge infection, no relevant pathological alterations were observed, other than enlarged mandibular and popliteal lymph nodes in a majority of cats from both groups, confirming the findings of the clinical examinations.

Although most cats did not develop severe symptoms linked to the challenge infection, 2 cats had to be euthanized at week 8 post-infection, due to early development of the AIDS phase of FIV disease. Cat I1 from the control group demonstrated enlarged mandibular and popliteal lymph nodes, severe gingivitis, glossitis, pharyngitis and conjunctivitis with purulent ocular discharge, accompanied by fever (41, 2°C body temperature), apathy and anorexia. Necropsy confirmed these clinical findings. Cat S3 from the dSLIM™-treated group was also euthanized, presenting high fever (41°C), anorexia and apathy. In this cat however, enlarged mandibular and popliteal lymph nodes were the only abnormal findings at necropsy.

5.2 Hematology

Red and white blood cell parameters were measured weekly in all cats. Unfortunately the hematological analysis carried out immediately before the onset of the experiment (w0-5d) revealed differences in the group mean values for a majority of parameters. These differences were however mainly non-significant and therefore not taken into consideration when interpreting the hematological alterations discussed below.

5.2.1 Red Blood Cell Parameters

Red blood cell (RBC) counts (figure 15), hemoglobin concentration, and mean cellular hemoglobin concentration (MCHC) indicated stable values in both groups throughout the experiment. Only the mean hematocrit values indicated a significant decline in the control group between time point of infection and week 2 post-challenge. Importantly, significant declines in mean hematocrit values were already observed for both groups during the treatment period, namely between the time points week 0-3d and week 0 (figure 16). No significant differences between both groups were noted for any RBC parameter during the entire duration of the experiment.

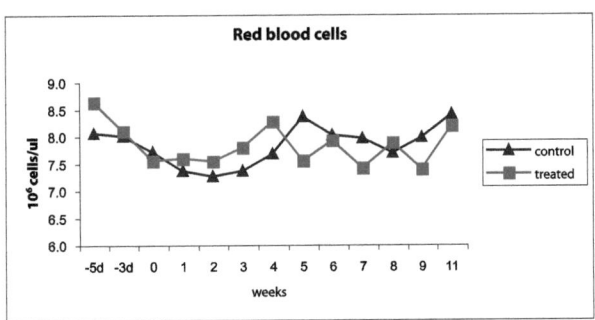

Figure 15: Mean red blood cell (RBC) counts (x10^6 cells/µl)

Results

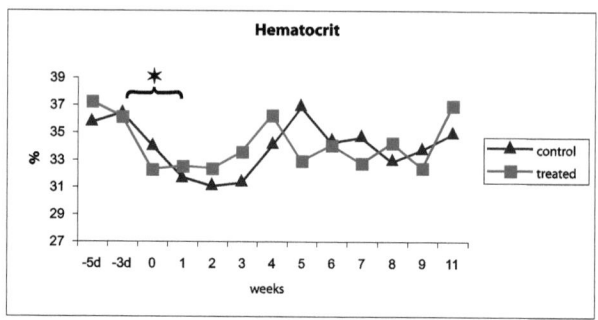

Figure 16: Mean hematocrit values (%)

5.2.2 White Blood Cell Parameters

5.2.2.1 Absolute White Blood Cell Counts

The absolute WBC counts measured in both groups indicated similar curves during the entire duration of the experiment. However, a significant peak in the values obtained for the dSLIM™-treated group at the time point week 0-3 days can be seen in figure 17. Although the graphic hints that the WBC values for the treated group stay well above those from the control group until week 2, these differences are not significant, due to high individual variability in the dSLIM™-treated group.

For both groups, the mean absolute WBC count decreased gradually between the time points of infection and euthanasia. More specifically, the drops observed in the first 2 weeks after FIV challenge are significant for both groups.

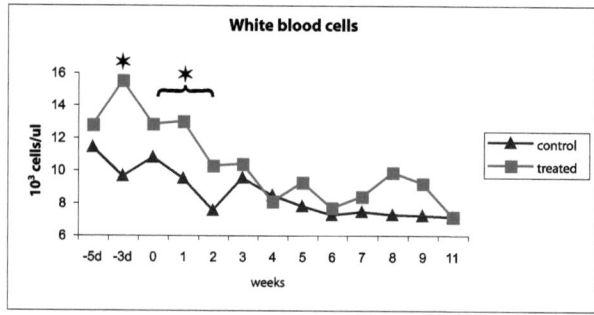

Figure 17: Mean white blood cell (WBC) counts (x10^3 cells /µl)

5.2.2.2 Neutrophilic and Eosinophilic Granulocytes

The graphical representation of the neutrophilic and eosinophilic granulocytes indicated curves similar to that of the mean WBC (figures 18 and 19). The mean values of both these parameters also decreased progressively and significantly during the entire duration of the experiment. Moreover, both during the treatment and immediately after challenge infection, increases in absolute counts of both neutrophilic and eosinophilic granulocytes were observed in the group treated with dSLIM™.

As illustrated in figure 18, the mean absolute neutrophil counts of the treated group peaked rapidly after the onset of the treatment (w0-3d). Both the peak in neutrophil count at week 0-3d, and the increase in mean values between week 0-5d and week 0-3d are significant. This rapid increase was due to neutrophilia in 4 individuals. Within a week's time after this peak however, the mean neutrophil count of the treated group dropped to similar values as the control group. Between weeks 3 and 6 after challenge infection, a highly significant decrease in neutrophils was observed in both groups. The decline in mean neutrophil count started earlier in the group of treated cats.

The particularly elevated mean levels of eosinophilic granulocytes until week 2 post-challenge (figure 19) are due to eosinophilia in 2 individuals from this group, thus rendering the divergence between the groups non-significant. However, as of week 2 after challenge infection, the eosinophil values of these cats returned to a normal range. The mean eosinophilc values for both groups hence indicate similar curves as of this time point.

Results

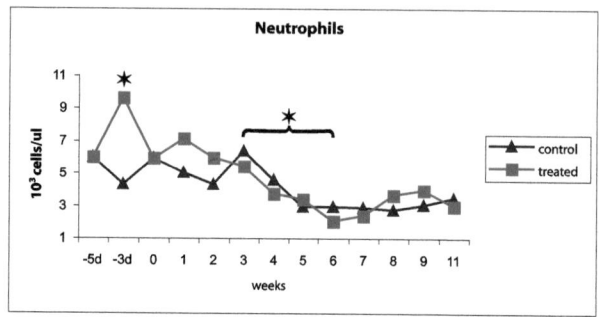

Figure 18: Mean absolute neutrophilic granulocyte counts (x10^3 cells /µl)

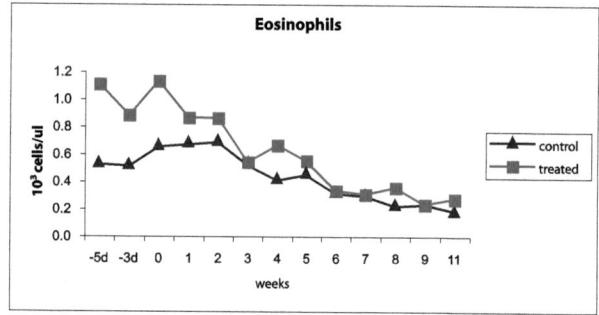

Figure 19: Mean absolute eosinophilic granulocyte counts (x103 cells /µl)

5.2.2.3 Monocytes

The dSLIM™-treated group displayed elevated mean absolute monocyte counts in comparison to the control group for mostly the entire duration of the study. However, due to high variability in the measured values between the individuals of this group, the differences were significant only at the beginning of the experiment, namely between the time points week 0-3 days and week 1 post challenge, as well as on week 9 (figure 20). The values measured in both groups always remained in the normal range.

Results

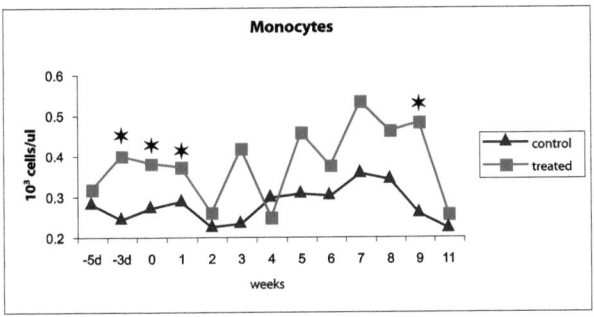

Figure 20: Mean absolute monocyte counts (x103 cells/µl)

5.2.2.4 Lymphocytes

A significant drop in mean lymphocyte values in both groups was due to a marked decrease in absolute lymphocyte counts and led to mild lymphopenia in most individuals of both groups within 2 weeks after challenge infection. Mean lymphocyte values regained normally expected levels by week 3 for the treated group and week 4 for the control group. Although the mean absolute lymphocyte counts of the treated group stayed below those of the control group during the entire duration of the study, the differences measured were not statistically significant (figure 21).

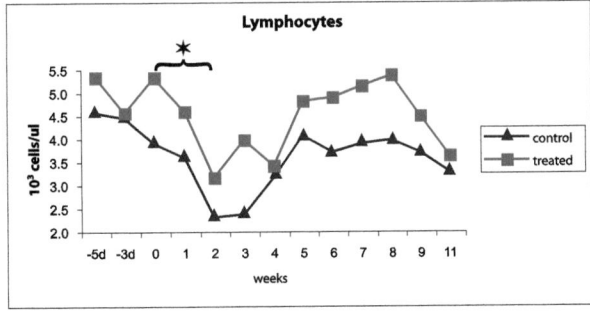

Figure 21: Mean absolute lymphocyte counts (x103 cells /µl)

137

Results

5.3 Clinical Chemistry

Although always comprised within a normal range, the mean values obtained for most parameters of clinical chemistry indicated divergences between the groups already before the onset of the study. As these differences were mainly non-significant, they were not taken into consideration when evaluating the results. The following sections highlight the significant differences encountered during analysis of the commonly tested substrates, enzymes and electrolytes in plasma.

5.3.1 Substrates

The blood glucose levels of the cats at the time of blood collections indicated many variations throughout the study. Moreover, in most individuals of the control group, hypoglycemic values were measured at the two first blood collections, and the differences between the groups at these time points were highly significant (p<0.01) (figure 22).

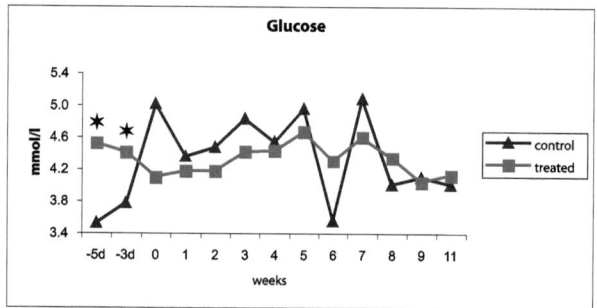

Figure 22: Mean blood glucose levels (mmol/l)

Additionally, elevated mean urea values in the treated group indicated highly significant differences between weeks 1 and 3 post challenge infection as well as at week 5, when compared to the control group (p< 0.01). Moreover, the urea levels of the treated cats indicate a significant increase between the time point of challenge and week 3 post-infection (figure 23).

All the other substrates analyzed in this study, namely bilirubin, creatinin, total protein, albumin and cholesterin concentrations indicated no significant divergences between both groups, or over time.

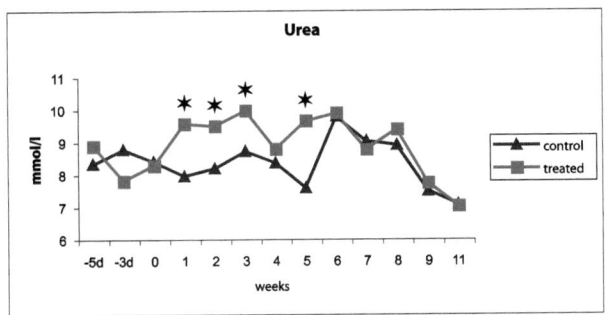

Figure 23: Mean blood urea levels (mmol/l)

5.3.2 Enzymes

Values for alanin-aminotransferase (ALAT), aspartate-aminotransferase (ASAT), alcaline phosphatase (AP) and lipase were evaluated weekly during this study. Interestingly, significant differences between the control group and the treated group were observed only for blood lipase values. The mean concentration of this enzyme in the plasma of the dSLIM™-treated cats indeed remained lower than that of the control cats for the entire study, with significance however only during the treatment period, that is 3 days before (w0-3d), and at the time point of challenge infection (w0) (figure 24).

Several individual cats sporadically demonstrated abnormally high levels of ALAT concentrations (> 100 U/l). This was the case for cat Q1 from the control group at weeks 8-9 post-infection. After FIV challenge, cats K3 and L4 from the treated group indicated similar transiently increased ALAT values at weeks 2 and 7-8 respectively (figure 25).

Results

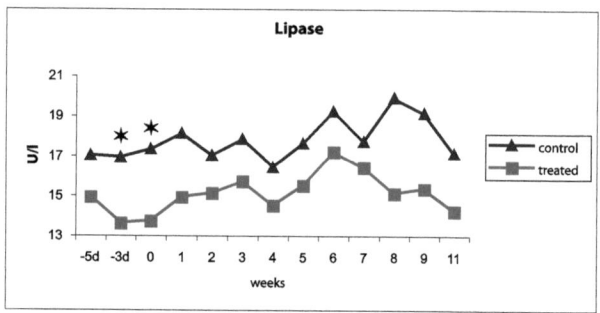

Figure 24: Mean blood lipase levels (U/l)

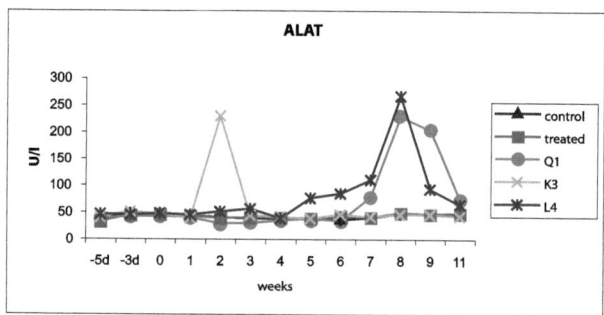

Figure 25: Mean blood alanin–aminotransferase (ALAT) levels (U/l). Values of cat Q1 from the control group and cats K3 and L4 from the treated group are illustrated separately.

5.3.3 Electrolytes

Although always comprised in the normal range, the mean concentrations of sodium, potassium, chloride and phosphate demonstrated considerable variability both within the groups and between the different weeks of the study. Significant alterations were however only observed for chloride and phosphate levels.

The chloride concentrations of both groups simultaneously increased slightly before challenge infection, and indicated a significant drop between weeks 0 and 1. The

Results

chloride concentrations in the treated group continued to decrease until week 2, inducing slight hypochloremia in most individuals of this group. However, by week 3, the values for both groups regained levels similar to those encountered before the treatment, and remained relatively stable for the rest of the study (figure 26).

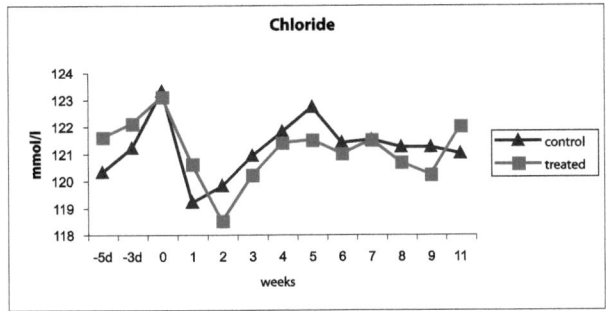

Figure 26: Mean blood chloride levels (mmol/l)

Both groups exhibited blood phosphorus values that were over the normal range for the entire experiment. However, phosphorus levels in the plasma of treated cats demonstrated significantly lower concentrations than the control group during the treatment period, and until week 1 post challenge infection (figure 27).

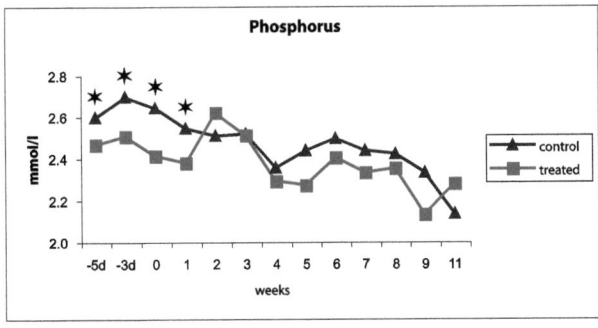

Figure 27: Mean blood phosphorus levels

Results

5.4 Immunology

5.4.1 Antibodies to FIV TM

In order to determine the time point of seroconversion and levels of antibodies to FIV developed over time after challenge infection, an anti-TM ELISA was carried out weekly. Low antibody levels were detected in most individuals of both groups already at week 1 and week 2 after FIV infection. By week 3 post-challenge, all cats had seroconverted and remained positive to ELISA until the end of the study. Generally, the results indicated two distinct peaks of antibody production after challenge infection, namely at weeks 5 and 7. These peaks were similar for both groups, although the mean antibody level of the treated group was higher than that of the control group at week 7. This difference was however not significant, in contrast to the divergences at weeks 3 and 8, time points at which the treated group displayed higher antibody levels than the control group (figure 28). The variability in antibody levels between individual cats was especially high between weeks 3 and 8 post challenge.

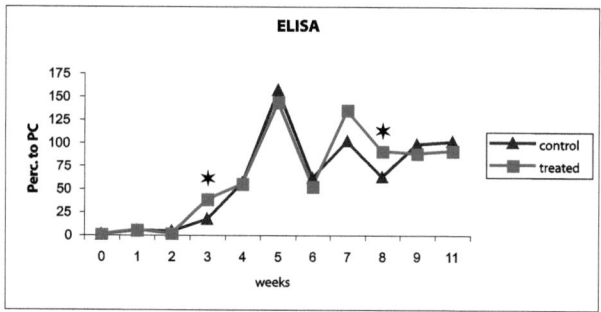

Figure 28: Mean serum anti-TM antibody levels, indicated using percentage of the positive control (Perc. to PC)

Importantly, 2 cats of the dSLIM™-treated group, M1 and T3, presented until week 4 post-challenge significantly lower antibody levels to FIV TM than the mean values measured for both the control group and treated group. These 2 cats also indicated

Results

a particularly favourable virological status during the acute phase of infection (see section 5.5).

5.4.2 Cytokine Measurements

Expression of GAPDH, IL-10 and IL-12 p40 was measured both in whole blood weekly, and in PBMCs isolated from the cats at 2 distinct time points during the experiment, namely on the day of challenge infection, and at week 8 post-challenge. As GAPDH is considered a «housekeeping» gene, the determination of a GAPDH:cytokine ratio enabled a standardization of the measurements obtained for IL-10 and IL-12 p40 during these experiments. This ratio is used as unit in the graphics illustrated in the following sections.

5.4.2.1 Cytokine Expression in Whole Blood

Measurement of IL-12 p40 and IL-10 expression in whole blood during treatment (w0-3d, w0-5d, w0) and after challenge (w1-w3,w7,w11)enabled to determine the expression kinetics of these cytokines throughout the study (figures 29-31).

Figure 29 reflects the mean quantitative results for GAPDH expression obtained in both groups. Only slight, non-significant divergences can be observed. However, both the drop between weeks 7 and 11 post-challenge in the treated group and the difference in expression levels of GAPDH between weeks 3 and 7 after FIV infection in the control group are significant.

The measured IL-10 mRNA expression levels throughout the study are demonstrated in figure 30. In both groups, no IL-10 expression could be detected during the entire duration of the treatment period. After challenge, IL-10 levels increased continuously in both groups until week 7, and decreased again to reach very low levels by week 11. As no measurements were carried out at weeks 8 and 9, it is not possible to determine both the maximal expression of IL-10, and how rapidly the

Results

expression levels effectively drop. The graphic indicates considerably lower levels of IL-10 for the treated group in comparison to the control group, especially at weeks 3 and 7 post-infection. As the results obtained for week 7 presented high individual variability in the control group, the latter findings are only significant at week 3.

In contrast to IL-10, IL-12 p40 was detectable during the treatment period. The measured expression levels indicate a higher increase post-infection in the control group than in the treated group. The augmentation in the control group of IL-12 p40 expression between weeks 0 and 2, along with the sudden drop between weeks 2 and 3, are both significant. However, between both groups, no significant differences could be measured throughout the whole study (figure 31).

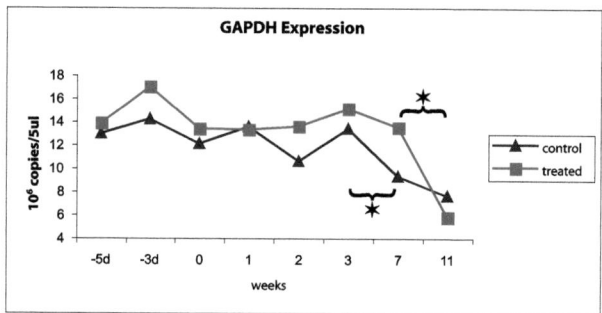

Figure 29: Mean GAPDH mRNA expression in whole blood (x10^6 copies/5μl)

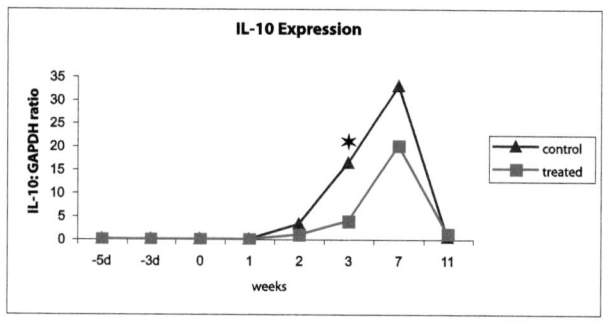

Figure 30: Mean IL-10 mRNA expression in whole blood (IL-10:GAPDH ratio)

Results

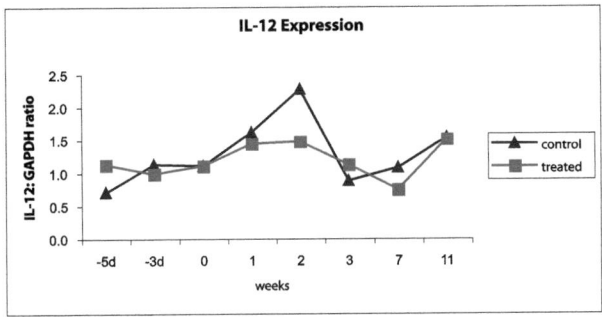

Figure 31: Mean IL-12 p40 mRNA expression in whole blood (IL-12: GAPDH ratio)

5.4.2.2 Stimulation of Cytokine Production *in vitro*

PBMCs were isolated from each cat individually twice during the course of the study, namely immediately before challenge infection (week 0), and at week 8 post-challenge, in order to evaluate the predominant cytokine expression pattern. Figures 32-34 illustrate the graphical results to these experiments.

Although the GAPDH graphics appear very similar at both time points analyzed, the columns representing the results for week 8 are shifted toward a lower level in comparison to those of week 0. Higher GAPDH levels were measured after Con A stimulation of PBMCs isolated from the cats of both groups, before, as well as after challenge infection.

Before challenge, i.e. at week 0, both the control and the treated group show no basal expression of IL-10, as is indicated by the measurements accomplished on the unstimulated PBMCs of the cats in both groups. However, at this time point, the expression of IL-10 by the lymphocytes of the control group was significantly increased in response to stimulation with Con A. A similar effect was encountered for the cells of the control group after LPS stimulation, although to lesser extent and lacking a significant difference to the treated cats. In contrast, at week 0, IL-10

Results

expression in PBMCs from treated cats could only be insignificantly stimulated by Con A, and not at all by LPS. Eight weeks after the challenge infection, only very low levels of IL-10 were measured in unstimulated PBMCs from both groups. When compared to the results obtained at week 0, the PBMCs isolated from the cats of the control group became significantly less responsive to Con A stimulation with regard to IL-10 mRNA levels. Lymphocytes from the treated cats expressed significantly higher IL-10 levels when stimulated with LPS 8 weeks after FIV challenge, than with the same stimulation before challenge, at week 0.

Although the basal IL-12 p40 expression measured in unstimulated PBMCs at week 0 was rather low in both groups, the immune cells from treated cats expressed significantly higher IL-12 p40 mRNA levels than those from control cats. Due to low variability in the obtained values, this difference is not obvious on the graph of figure 34. It is however indicated by a star. Similarly in both groups at week 0, stimulation of PBMCs with Con A and LPS enhanced expression of IL-12 p40 significantly. LPS stimulation thereby indicated far more potency in this effect. There was however no significance in the differences between the groups in IL-12 p40 expression levels after stimulation with Con A or LPS at this time point. Unstimulated PBMCs from the cats in both groups indicated significantly enhanced expression of IL-12 p40 at week 8 post-challenge, when compared to values obtained at week 0. However, the differences between both groups were thereby not significant. With respect to IL-12 p40 expression at week 8, the PBMCs from the control group are significantly more responsive to LPS stimulation, whereas those from the treated group are significantly less reactive to LPS stimulation, in comparison to the results of the same experiments accomplished at week 0. When mean mRNA levels of IL-12 p40 from both groups were compared at week 8, no significant differences were measured.

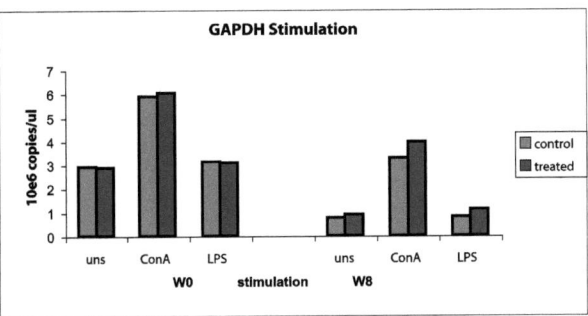

Figure 32: Mean GAPDH mRNA expression of isolated PBMCs from all cats in both groups, either 1) left unstimulated, 2) stimulated with ConA, or 3) stimulated with LPS ($\times 10^6$ copies/µl). Experiments were carried out at the time point of challenge (W0) and 8 weeks post-challenge (W8).

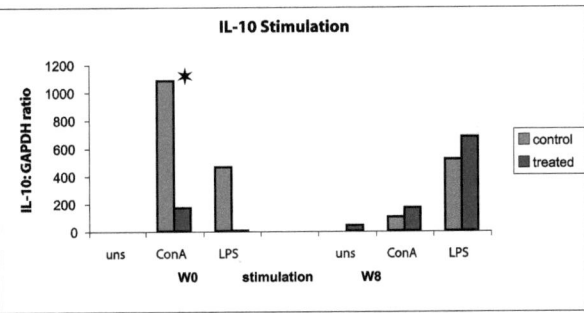

Figure 33: Mean IL-10 mRNA expression of isolated PBMCs from all cats in both groups, either 1) left unstimulated, 2) stimulated with ConA, or 3) stimulated with LPS (IL-10:GAPDH ratio). Experiments were carried out at the time point of challenge (W0) and 8 weeks post-challenge (W8).

Results

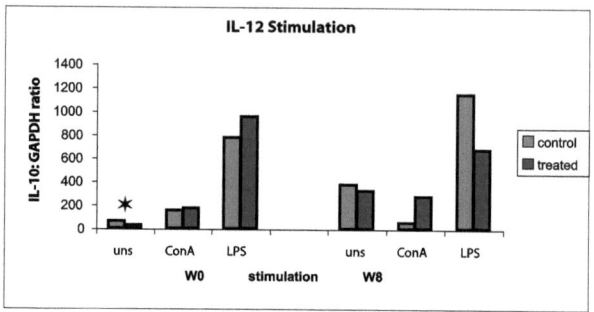

Figure 34: Mean IL-12 p40 mRNA expression of isolated PBMCs from all cats in both groups, either 1) left unstimulated, 2) stimulated with ConA, or 3) stimulated with LPS (IL-12:GAPDH ratio). Experiments were carried out at the time point of challenge (W0) and 8 weeks post-challenge (W8).

5.5 Evaluation of Viral Infection

5.5.1 FIV Proviral Loads in Whole Blood

FIV proviral load in peripheral blood cells was assessed weekly by real-time PCR analysis of TNA extracted from whole blood samples. Throughout the entire duration of the study, no significant differences in proviral loads between the groups were measured. In a similar manner for both groups, the proviral loads rapidly increased until week 3 and remained relatively stable until the end of the study. With the exception of week 2, the CT values obtained for the treated group remained slightly higher than those of the control group until week 4. Moreover, although presence of FIV infection could be assessed in all cats of the control group at weeks 1 to 3 post-challenge, 2 cats of the dSLIM™-treated group, M1 and T3, remained provirus negative by real-time PCR until week 4 after FIV challenge (figure 35). Although the individual proviral loads for these 2 cats stay below those of the control group between weeks 5 and 11 post-infection by a factor of more than 15-fold, these differences are not significant.

Results

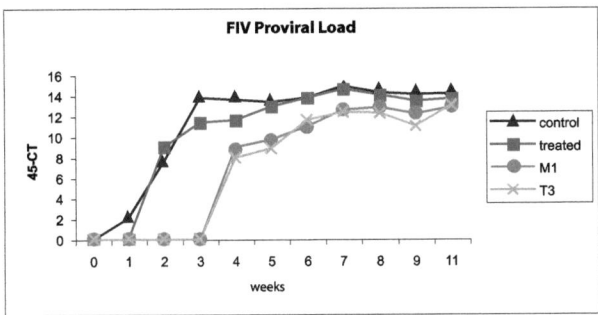

Figure 35: Mean FIV proviral loads in whole blood (45-CT values). Values for cats M1 and T3 from the treated group are illustrated seperately.

Interestingly, in the cats I1 and S3, which had to be euthanized at the 8th week after FIV challenge, the proviral load had increased rapidly in the acute phase of infection and remained particularly high throughout the experiment. The difference between the proviral kinetics of these 2 individuals and those of the respective mean group values was however not significant (data not shown).

5.5.2 FIV Viral Load

5.5.2.1 FIV Viral Load in Plasma

FIV viral load in plasma was measured weekly by real-time RT-PCR analysis. In both groups, the measured viral loads increased rapidly until week 2 post-challenge, similarly to the previously discussed proviral loads. In contrast to the latter however, the mean viral loads in plasma diminish gradually until the end of the study. No significant differences between the 2 groups were observed at any time point throughout the experiment. Also, the 2 cats euthanized at week 8 post-challenge presented viral RNA levels in plasma which corresponded to the mean group values throughout the experiment.

Results

Importantly, no viral RNA was measured in the plasma of 2 cats, M1 and T3 until week 4 after challenge with FIV. These individuals equally remained provirus negative until this time point (see above: 5.5.1). Although at week 4 post-infection the viral loads detected in the plasma of M1 and T3 were not yet quite as high as those from both groups, this difference was not significant, and the loads measured onward were similar to the means of the control group and treated group values (figure 36).

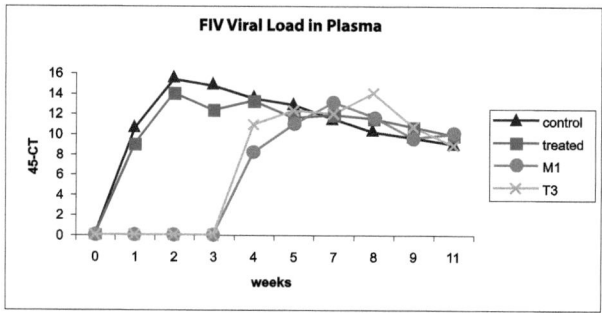

Figure 36: Mean FIV viral loads in plasma (45-CT values). Values for cats M1 and T3 from the treated group are illustrated seperately.

5.5.2.2 FIV Viral Load in Saliva

FIV viral loads in saliva obtained from the collection of buccal swabs were measured on a weekly basis by real-time RT-PCR. For both groups, 2 peaks of viral secretion in saliva were observed at weeks 5 and 9 post-infection. During the 11 weeks of the study, no significant differences with respect to FIV shedding in saliva were observed between the groups. However, during both peaks, namely at weeks 5 and 9 post-infection, the treated group seemingly demonstrated slightly higher mean viral loads in saliva, which was due not only to viral secretion by more individuals at these time points, but also to shedding of higher amounts of virus by these individuals in comparison to the control group (figures 37 and 38).

The 2 cats from the treated group, which presented negative proviral and viral loads until week 3 post-challenge infection, displayed diverging results: cat M1 secreted virus in saliva as of week 9 post-infection, whereas no FIV RNA could be measured in the saliva of cat T3 during the entire study. Interestingly, both cats which had to be euthanized at week 8 after challenge infection did not secrete virus in their saliva during the entire experiment.

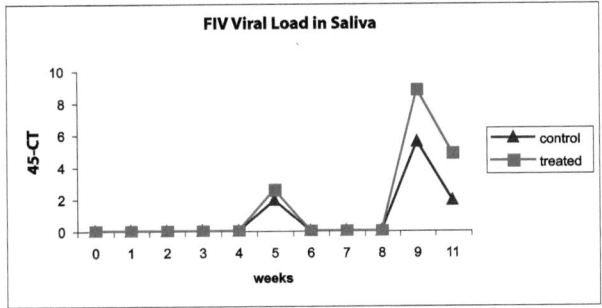

Figure 37: Mean FIV viral loads in saliva (45-CT value)

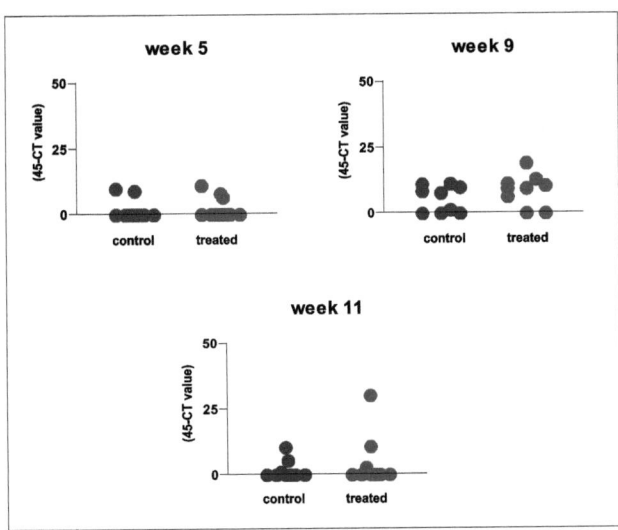

Figure 38: Individual FIV viral loads in saliva of all cats for weeks 5, 9, 11 (45-CT values). No virus was detected in any cat on weeks 0,1,2,3,4,6,7 (graphs not shown).

Results

5.5.3 Isolation of Virus from Plasma

Presence of infectious virus in plasma was evaluated by a cell culture inoculation method weekly between weeks 2 and 8 post-challenge. Real-time RT-PCR of culture supernatants revealed for both groups a similar peak of infectious virus release in plasma at week 4. Although presence of infectious virus could be demonstrated in the plasma of 6 treated cats and 8 control cats on week 2 post-infection, it could only be detected in 1 treated cat and 7 control cats on week 3 post-challenge, rendering the difference at this time point significant. At week 8 post-infection however, infectious virus could be isolated from plasma of all cats of the treated group, but only from 8 cats of the control group. This difference is also significant, to the benefit of the control group (figure 39). Between weeks 2 and 7 after FIV challenge infection, the mean amount of infectious virus isolated from plasma of the treated cats stayed slightly lower than that of control cats (data not shown).

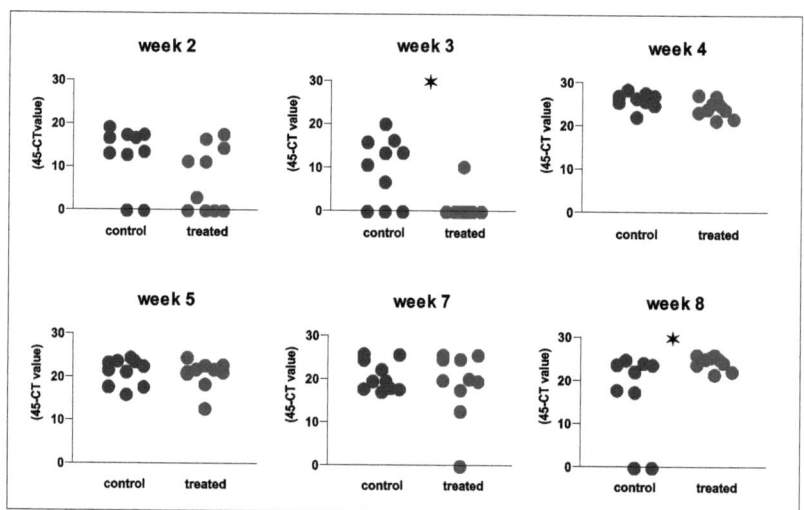

Figure 39: Infectious FIV isolation from all cats on weeks 2,3,4,5,7,8 after challenge infection (45-CT values, with individual CT values measured in supernatants of PBMC cultures)

Cats M1 and T3 from the dSLIM™-treated group became viremic at week 4 after FIV infection (see 5.5.2.1), and started producing infectious virus rapidly thereafter. Indeed, no infectious virus could be isolated from the PBMCs of these individuals in weeks 2 and 3 post-challenge, but both indicated production of infectious virus as of the week 4 post-infection in quantities comparable to all other cats in the study.

6. Discussion

6.1 Background of the study

It was the aim of this study to stimulate the innate immune system of the domestic cat with a synthetic, CpG-containing molecule and induce short term prophylactic resistance to a challenge infection with FIV. Clinical and immunopathological parameters of the cats were closely monitored during the acute phase of infection in order to assess any indication of resistance to FIV infection or disease. We expected to observe an innate immune response capable of either preventing or delaying 1) establishment of infection in the host's immune cells, 2) progression to viremia and secretion of infectious virus in saliva, or 3) onset or severity of clinical symptoms linked to FIV infection. Capability of conferring only partial resistance to domestic cats against FIV in this study was to be considered as partial success. Prophylactic induction of innate immunity is a relatively novel idea, and such findings would open new unexplored paths in preventive medicine in both human and veterinary fields.

A pet cat temporarily placed in a cattery or shelter rarely goes back home entirely healthy. Narrow contact of cats from totally different backgrounds in such establishments creates an environment highly favorable for transmission of various feline viral diseases. Common known feline viruses indeed possess both very efficient transmission strategies and the capability to induce latent and/or asymptomatic infections of the carrier cat. These properties were hypothetically gained over thousands of years by viruses adapted to the feline host, in order to survive in a population with a very solitary way of life, probably due to restricted food basis. Although modern civilization, starting with the domestication by man of cattle, sheep and goats around 5000 years ago, provides the food basis allowing

Discussion

cats to live in groups, feline viruses have conserved their opportunistic behaviour. Regroupment of cats in facilities such as agricultural farms, shelters and catteries considerably increases the infectious pressure. Also, in shelters for example, the animals' immune systems are already sensitized by the stress conferred by a new environment populated with unknown individuals, which additionally favours susceptibility to infectious agents. As the onset of disease caused by these viruses is often delayed, infection of their cats frequently remains unnoticed by the owners for long periods of time. Not only symptoms usually appear in advanced stages of disease, when it becomes difficult to cure, but this time span may enable the virus to disseminate in new hosts. Unfortunately, owing to the adaptation properties of feline viruses, elaboration of effective preventive and therapeutic methods has proven to be particularly challenging. The cat is one of the most appreciated companion animals worldwide, and catteries and shelters are widely established in the developed countries. In the interest of both the owners and of entire populations of pet cats, it would be highly desirable to have an effective antiviral agent available, which would, on the occasion of regroupment of cats for a short period of time, confer the host resistance to a broad spectrum of viral diseases. Moreover, the use of broad spectrum antiviral agents could be extrapolated to other animals or to humans, as new emerging viral diseases currently constitute a constant threat of pandemic to these populations.

Inspired by a need in the veterinary medical field, the design of this study was based on a modern scientific background. Better understanding the complexity of the innate immune system has been a major subject of the last 10 to 15 years in medical biology. It became rapidly clear that stimulation of the organism's first line of defence could be exploited to enhance resistance to a variety of infections. Stimulation of innate immunity not only initiates immediate reaction to a wide range of pathogens, but greatly supports the subsequent development of a specific immune response, representing a feasible alternative method to specific immunization. Since the complex network of interactions between the cells involved in the organism's first line of defence represents a phylogenetically ancient form of immune response,

Discussion

the molecular participants of innate immunity are encoded in the genome of the host and have been conserved throughout evolution. It is today widely accepted, that early pathogen recognition of the innate immune system relies on its ability to recognize microbial components known as PAMPs [223]. These molecules are essential for the survival of the microorganisms and therefore only rarely alter in the course of evolution.

Many research groups have concentrated in recent years on the development of synthetic versions of PAMPs and on their testing as new pharmaceutical products in various disease settings. CpG ODNs are among the most thoroughly studied PAMPs. The innate immune system of fish, birds and mammals efficiently recognize and respond to bacterial DNA because it contains, in contrast to vertebrate DNA, a high amount of unmethylated CpG motifs. Recognition of CpG motifs is considered an ancient defence mechanism of the vertebrates against invading pathogens and its evolutionary conservation over tens of millions of years strongly indicates that CpG-mediated immune activation contributes to host survival. Feasibility of experiments with CpG-containing molecules is furthermore supported by the ease in production and modulation of synthetic CpG ODNs. Several generations of ODN structures, containing variable numbers and flanking sequences of CpG motifs, have been designed and tested, thus allowing the development of highly potent immunomodulators capable of targeting specific elements of the immune system. Moreover, although response to CpG motifs was originally predestined for early combat against bacterial infection, exposure of immune cells to natural or synthetic CpG-containing molecules generally triggers the creation of an immune environment highly favourable to antiviral mechanisms, comprising deviation to cellular responses as well as liberation of Th1-derived cytokines and considerable amounts of IFN-α [283]. This type I IFN is known for its capacity to induce, in yet uninfected cells, the expression of various proteins including enzymes, signaling proteins, antigen presenting proteins and transcription factors, which directly interfere with viral replication and thus establish an intracellular antiviral state [377]. Considering the immunopotency of CpG ODNs, a carefully selected synthetic compound containing CpG motifs thus appeared optimal for the mounting of an

Discussion

immune response capable of competing with viral challenge in the cat.

Among the most common feline viruses, FIV appeared to be the most reasonable choice of challenge when experimenting the prophylactic properties of CpG ODNs. Both the elevated worldwide prevalence of this persistent lethal infection in populations of domestic cats and the lack of an appropriate vaccine and effective therapeutic agents on the market pressure development of novel strategies to diminish dissemination of the disease. Investigations on the genes of the lentivirus subfamily of retroviruses, including HIV, SIV, FIV, equine infectious anemia (EIAV) and ovine lentivirus Visna have indicated comparatively extremely low frequencies of CpG dinucleotides in their DNA [378]. Boosting the defence mechanisms elicited by CpG motifs may help compensate the insufficient natural stimulation of this immune pathway and therefore appeared especially feasible in the context of such infections. Moreover, FIV appeared especially sensitive to IFN-α in several studies, considerably increasing chances that immunomodulatory effects of CpG ODNs could contribute efficiently to the mounting of resistance to FIV infection [61, 175]. Finally, FIV infection in the cat is considered a close model of HIV in humans [57], and such experiments may reveal precious information on various biological and immunopathological properties of these retroviruses and open the way to unexplored paths in HIV research.

6.2 Design of the Study

The design of the present experiment involved preliminary determination of important parameters, which are discussed below.

In order to improve reliability of the results obtained, high importance was attributed to provenance, amount, age, gender, and health status of the cats used for the study. The experiment was accomplished with 20 spf cats, divided into 2 groups of 10 cats each. We have chosen to utilize the minimal amount of individuals enabling to determine significant divergences which would have future clinical relevance.

Discussion

Moreover, all cats were ordered from a specialized facility breeding domestic cats under spf conditions, and the perfect health of the animals was ensured through professional examination by a veterinarian at their arrival. Influence of the genetic background of the cats on the reactions linked to the treatment was considerably diminished by selecting cats from different litters and with different parents. Also, as the immune system of young cats is more prone to react to various stimuli, kittens of approximately 2 months of age were requested. Finally, to increase accuracy when comparing parameters measured throughout the experiment, balanced distribution of the individuals into the two groups was considered crucial. Thus, the cats were divided in the groups according to litter provenance and age, and we insisted on receiving only male cats. To avoid risks of bias in attribution of individuals to the respective groups, the distribution was effected blindly before the arrival of the cats. Unfortunately, certain cats turned out to be considerably smaller than the others despite similar birth dates, and significant differences in the mean body weights were measured between both groups already before the onset of the experiment. This is probably the explanation for the slight divergences observed early in the study in many hematological and biological parameters tested in the cats. As this data confers important indications on side effects or pathological alterations, greater value should be attributed to similar average body weights in both groups at the start of future experiments.

Treatment of the cats was performed with dSLIM™, a carefully selected molecule with multiple advantages for the present study. First, this non-coding DNA molecule contains several unmethylated CpG motifs and possesses the broad spectrum immunomodulatory properties of Class C CpG ODNs. Thus, dSLIM™ is capable of simultaneously mobilizing many different components of the immune system [379]. Secondly, dSLIM™ is protected *in vivo* from destruction by cellular nucleases through its special covalently-closed, dumbbell shape. This configuration not only confers dSLIM™ high stability when administered in the host, but represents a feasible alternative to synthesis of the molecule with a phosphorothioate backbone, known to induce many undesired side effects when

Discussion

applied *in vivo*. Finally, immunomodulatory effects and safety of dSLIM™ have been systematically demonstrated in both *in vitro* and *in vivo* studies, in humans, non-human primates, dogs and mice, indicating efficacy in many species [374, 380]. Moreover, this molecule has indicated such promising results that it is currently being clinically trialed in various human disease settings [381].

The administration protocol of dSLIM™ was adjusted to published facts on duration and extent of immunomodulation by CpG ODNs. The innate immune response elicited by CpG DNA was previously shown to peak within days and promote effective defence mechanisms within the host for about 2 weeks [359]. Also, repeated administration of CpG ODNs as stand-alone protective agent was shown to maintain the host's resistance to infection [382]. Finally, administration of CpG ODNs by many different routes, including i.v., i.m., i.p., s.c., p.o. have indicated systemic immunostimulation. Thus, the cats were treated using a combination of administration methods over a period of 5 consecutive days. The combination of s.c, i.p and i.v administration of dSLIM™ favored a broad *in vivo* distribution. Moreover, subcutaneous injections of dSLIM™ were specially foreseen to activate a maximal amount of dentritic cells present in the layers of the skin. As the challenge infection was accomplished i.p, it seemed reasonable to include this mode of administration, in order to enable accumulation of dSLIM™ at the site of infection. The combination of several modes of administration in the same *in vivo* experiment however prevents from determining which is the most successful. We were aware that further experiments would be necessary to determine the optimal route of injection in the cat. Additionally, five consecutive days of treatment enabled to potentiate the immunostimulatory effects of dSLIM™ for the time point of challenge, which took place 24 hours after the end of the treatment, and for the acute phase of infection, when the host's immune status highly influences the future outcome of disease.

The challenge infection is another determining factor in the outcome of the experiment. The cats were challenged i.p., widely accepted to be the mode of administration of the virus which best mimics natural infection. Also, the time point

Discussion

of challenge infection was selected according to the time when optimal host defence mechanisms stimulated by the treatment were anticipated. FIV-GL8, used for the challenge infection in this experiment, is known to be a particularly virulent strain. However, the viral stock utilized had previously been titrated *in vivo* by another laboratory, and the lowest titre effectively infecting 100% of the cats was chosen, both ensuring reliability in interpretation of the prophylactic effects induced by the treatment, and leaving space for the observation of the slightest effects. As several vaccine studies [189, 214] have previously indicated that FIV-GL8 seems more resistant to vaccinal immunity than other known FIV strains, this type of challenge may have been too aggressive in the context of unspecific host defence mechanisms. However, in consideration of these facts, we measured a broad selection of immunological parameters in the cats during the course of the study, thus analyzing several levels of the viral-host interactions, and increasing the chances to observe hints of resistance to FIV infection. Also, the elaboration of a preventive measure against a virulent strain is particularly challenging, and promising results would reveal solid optimism for its clinical application.

For several reasons, we have decided to test the prophylactic effect of dSLIM™ directly *in vivo*. As already mentioned, it is a common property of all vertebrates to have acquired throughout evolution the capability to recognize and respond to CpG ODNs. Detailed studies have shown that the innate immune system of many out-bred domestic and non-domestic animals respond to the same CpG-containing DNA sequences [260, 296]. Moreover, in recent years, great scientific interest in this field has enabled the development of highly specific molecules as well as their testing in a wide variety of species *in vitro* and *in vivo*. Finally, many physiological and immunological parameters which greatly influence the success of a prophylactic agent cannot be taken into consideration when tested *in vitro*. Unfortunately, despite thorough preparation and realization of the experiment, the immunopathlogical and virological parameters evaluated did not indicate significant resistance against infection or disease in the treated group. Previous *in vitro* optimization of dSLIM™ would have permitted a more precise prediction and modulation of the *in vivo*

Discussion

experiment. Moreover, as the risk of acceleration of retroviral disease development has been described in earlier studies and attributed to the replication-enhancing effect of virus target cell populations by the treatment [331, 340], an *in vitro* testing of dSLIM™ on feline peripheral blood immune cells would have enabled to more surely exclude the risk of such an occurrence. This fact will be seriously considered for future experiments.

Nevertheless, interesting findings in this study may shed light on various aspects of the pathogenesis and immunoprophylaxy of FIV disease, as well as on the use of CpG ODNs in the feline species. These issues are discussed in further detail below.

6.3 Relevant Results

6.3.1 Results of the Clinical Examinations

In order to enable an accurate follow-up of the clinical status of each individual, examinations of the cats were carried out weekly, and always by the same veterinarian. In this way, important clinical findings, such as number of enlarged lymph nodes and grade of enlargement, could be somewhat standardized. Although this was not a blind study, great importance was attributed to the objective assessment of the cats' health conditions.

The present study represents the first evaluation of the effects of dSLIM™ *in vivo* in the cat. Thus, it appeared imperative to closely examine the cats for any signs of undesired side effects or toxicity caused by the treatment, and to assess any specific indication of intolerance to the different routes of administration of dSLIM™. Safety concerns linked to the administration of CpG ODNs *in vivo* have been mostly depicted after either particularly high dosage, repeated administration in short intervals over several weeks or months, or phosphorothioate modification of the DNA backbone. Previously described symptoms include general apathy and discomfort, excessive bleeding due to prolonged blood clotting time, splenomegaly,

Discussion

autoimmune diseases and toxic shock as a result of over-production of TNF-α [292-294]. The choice of dSLIM™ as immunomodulatory agent considerably minimized the risk of encountering such adverse reactions in this study. Quantities and frequency of dSLIM™ administration were derived and adjusted from dosage protocols used in human clinical trials. Also, the configuration of dSLIM™ protects this molecule enough from cellular nucleases to avoid the need of a phosphorothioate backbone. However, as dSLIM™ is known to induce enhanced production of IL-6, a potent pro-inflammatory cytokine, special attention was attributed to body temperature of the cats during treatment. The mean body temperatures of the treated group surprisingly remained lower than those of the control group during the treatment period, and no individuals had fever during the treatment. The cats were also methodically checked for indications of local toxicity, allergy or inflammation at the site of injection. Regardless of the mode of administration, no local or systemic adverse reactions obviously linked to the treatment with dSLIM™ were observed during the entire experiment.

Since FIV-GL8 is known to be a particularly virulent strain, it was expected that at least the control cats would exhibit early, marked symptoms of acute infection and/or rapid progression to AIDS-related disease. Typical symptoms of acute FIV infection, mainly slight apathy and enlargement of palpable lymph nodes, were recognized in all cats between weeks 3 and 6 post-challenge. Neither more rapid onset of disease nor more pronounced symptoms were observed in the control cats in comparison to the treated individuals. Moreover, one cat in each group had to be euthanized for ethical reasons at week 8 after FIV challenge. Both animals demonstrated apathy and particularly high fever. These symptoms were accompanied by severe, typical symptoms of AIDS-related disease in the cat belonging to the control group. As the immunomodulatory effects of CpG ODN administration *in vivo* have been shown to last no longer than a few weeks, it is highly unlikely that the further development of disease would have differed between the groups if we had extended the experiment. The particularly bad clinical state and the pathological findings at necropsy of one cat in the control group are insufficient indications of more rapid

Discussion

disease progression in this group. These facts altogether indicate that dSLIM™ unfortunately failed to confer even partial protection from disease in this study.

6.3.2 Blood Parameters

Both haematological status and parameters of clinical chemistry were systematically evaluated during this study. These examinations permitted to 1) keep a valuable overview on the health status of the animals during the entire duration of the study, 2) screen any hematologic or metabolic abnormalities linked to treatment with dSLIM™ and 3) characterize the hematosuppressive effects of FIV-GL8 infection as well as the extent of possible secondary affections.

Unfortunately the analyses of parameters of haematology and clinical chemistry carried out immediately before the onset of the experiment (w0-5d) revealed differences in the group mean values of a majority of parameters. This is probably due to the distribution of the cats in the groups according to age and not to body weight. Although mainly non-significant, these differences unfortunately complicate the interpretation of the data. The main divergences encountered during the study regarding these parameters are nevertheless discussed below.

6.3.2.1 Haematology

6.3.2.1.1 Deviation in Red Blood Cell Parameters

6.3.2.1.1.1 Hematocrit

The hematosuppressive effects induced by retroviral infection may include mild to moderate anemia in the acute phase of infection [383]. Thus, the temporary and significant decrease in the mean hematocrit values of the control group was probably linked to the challenge with FIV. Interestingly, the mean values for this parameter remained relatively stable in the treated group after infection.

Discussion

The collection of 3 times 4ml of blood with a period of 5 days is mostly to be the cause of the significant decline in mean hematocrit values observed during the treatmet period between both groups.

6.3.2.1.2. Deviation in White Blood Cell Parameters

6.3.2.1.2.1 Leucocytes

Although both groups exhibited a significant decrease in mean absolute leucocyte counts during the first 2 weeks after challenge, the values obtained in this experiment did not comply with the previously described acute phase leucopenia in FIV infection [146]. However, the drop in leucocyte counts mentioned above, as well as the subsequent gradual decrease observed during the rest of the study, are most likely related to infection with FIV.

During the treatment period and until week 2 post-infection, higher average leucocyte values were measured for the treated group, with significance only on the third day of treatment. All the other subpopulations of white blood cells measured for the treated group in this study, namely neutrophilic and eosinophilic granulocytes, lymphocytes and monocytes, indicated simultaneously increased absolute counts. The proliferation of these cell populations will be discussed in more detail in the corresponding sections below, enabling a better interpretation of the observed augmentation in leucocytes.

6.3.2.1.2.2 Neutrophilic Granulocytes

In a similar way to those of the total WBC, the mean neutrophil counts of the control group shortly increased two weeks after challenge infection, and decreased rapidly between the third and sixth week post-infection. This finding has already been described and has been related to FIV infection [384]. Interestingly, the same pattern appeared 2 weeks in advance for the treated group.

Discussion

The mean neutrophil counts of the treated group were influenced by neutrophilia in four individuals 3 days after the onset of the treatment. The recruitment of non-circulating neutrophils in these cats may be due to induction of an inflammatory environment by the administration of dSLIM™, known to increase production of IL-6, or to a particularly high level of stress during that blood collection.

6.3.2.1.2.3 Eosinophilic Granulocytes

As dSLIM™ was shown to be a potent mediator of Th1 immune responses, proliferation of eosinophils was not expected in the treated group. Indeed, this eosinophil activation is commonly linked to a Th2 immune environment, which should be suppressed by the effects of dSLIM™. However, two cats of the treated group presented considerable eosinophilia during the treatment period and until shortly after infection. As these individuals already presented high eosinophil values before the onset of the experiment, the observed alterations cannot be considered a consequence of the treatment. The return to normal values in these 2 cats as of week 2 post-infection remains unclear.

6.3.2.1.2.4 Monocytes

The cats from the treated group showed higher levels of monocytes during the treatment, and until week 1 post-challenge infection. Moreover, until the end of the study, the mean monocyte values for this group remained slightly higher than those of the control group. The divergences between both groups for this parameter were surprisingly greater than in all the other white blood cell subpopulations ($p<0.007$). Thus, treatment with dSLIM™ seemingly activated proliferation or circulation of monocytes in the cats. Interestingly, direct activation of this cell population with CpG ODNs has been described only in experiments with mice [365]. Human monocytes, in contrast, lack expression of TLR9, and the observed activation of this white blood cell type has been attributed to the effects of phosphorothioate backbones [271]. These facts taken into consideration, the activation of monocytes

Discussion

in cats after administration of dSLIM™ observed during the present study is rather surprising. Indeed, as most species respond in a similar manner to CpG ODNs, it was suggested that the divergences observed in several murine experiments could be in relation to the inbreeding of these animals. Moreover, the dSLIM™ molecule contains no phosphorothioate or other synthetic modifications. Further experiments would be required to both determine whether feline monocytes express TLR9, and to characterize the molecular and cellular mechanisms linked to this activation.

6.3.2.1.2.5 Lymphocytes

Most individuals from both groups demonstrated a significant drop in lymphocyte counts immediately after FIV infection leading to mild lymphopenia by week 2 post-challenge, but returning to normal values shortly. Lymphopenia more commonly characterizes chronic, symptomatic FIV disease. However, a mild, temporary lymphopenia, similar to that encountered in acute HIV and SIV infections, has also been described in the acute phase of FIV infection [125].

Mean lymphocyte counts of the treated group remained slightly higher than those of the control group throughout the whole study. However, this difference was already measured before the onset of the study, and the divergences lacked significance during the whole experiment, rendering the interpretation of this finding particularly difficult. As CpG ODNs are known to activate B lymphocytes and NK cells directly, as well as T lymphocytes indirectly, it was initially expected to observe an increase in absolute lymphocyte counts in the treated cats [289].

6.3.2.2 Clinical Chemistry

6.3.2.2.1 Substrates

6.3.2.2.1.2 Blood Glucose Levels

The blood glucose levels of the cats at the time of blood collections vary considerably

Discussion

throughout the entire study. Moreover, during the treatment period, hypoglycaemic values were measured in many individuals of the control group, leading to highly significant differences when compared to the normal values of the treated cats. This significance was however already observed in the measurements carried out immediately before the onset of the treatment. Thus, it is unlikely that dSLIM™ played a role in this observation. As kittens lack fat reserves, they are particularly susceptible to hypoglycemia when not fed regularly. The cats from both groups were fed several times a day in similar quantities adapted to their physiological needs. Moreover, in order to both diminish time between two meals and avoid vomiting and aspiration risks during sedation, the blood collections always took place early in the morning. The cats were systematically fed as late as possible the night before, namely about 12 hours prior to the administration of the sedatives. For organization purposes, the blood collections always took place with the control group first, then carried on with the treated group. Thus, lower blood glucose levels were accordingly expected in the treated cats, as this group was left to fast for a couple more hours than the control group. The slight differences in mean body weight from both groups at the beginning of the study is unlikely to be the reason for this observation, since the treated group contained a greater amount of small individuals and was constrained to longer durations of fasting. Although stress factors could be an explanation for increased blood glucose levels in cats, stressed animals commonly indicate hyperglycemia, which was not the case for the individuals in the treated group. It is important to mention here that as the time between blood collections and measurements was inferior to 2 hours, the use of fluoride tubes did not seem necessary in this experiment; this strategy will however be considered in future experiments.

Altogether, the reasons for the state of hypoglycaemia in the kittens of the control group, and the meaning of the highly significant differences between both groups during the treatment period remain difficult to explain.

6.3.2.2.1.3 Blood Urea Levels

A significant increase in mean blood urea levels was observed immediately after FIV challenge in the treated group, and elevated blood urea values induced highly significant differences between the groups between weeks 1 and 3 post challenge as well as at week 5. Since blood creatinin values were normal in all cats during the entire experiment, alterations in the kidneys could be excluded. As all cats received the same quantity and the same brand of food, this was unlikely to an influencing factor. These observations may indicate a delayed effect of dSLIM™ treatment on protein metabolism. However, it is difficult to say whether this effect is linked to or influenced by the challenge infection.

6.3.2.2.2 Enzymes

6.3.2.2.2.1 Lipase

Significantly lower lipase values were measure in the blood of the treated cats during treatment period. However, the lipase levels measured immediately before the onset of treatment were also lower in this group, than in the control group. Although the difference at this time point was not significant, it renders the interpretation of these findings rather difficult, and the explanation for these divergences remains unclear.

6.3.2.2.2.2 ALAT

One individual cat in the control group and two from the treated group sporadically demonstrated abnormally high levels of ALAT concentrations, most likely indicating transitory liver alterations. This observation is most likely due to individual responses to FIV challenge infection. Surprisingly, both cats euthanized at week 8 post infection (I1 and S3) had normal ALAT values for the entire duration of the study, including when they developed FIV disease.

Discussion

6.3.2.2.3 Electrolytes

6.3.2.2.3.1 Blood Chloride Levels

The simultaneous highly significant decrease in blood chloride concentrations immediately after challenge infection, leading to hypochloremia in both groups within two weeks, remains unclear. No symptoms of vomiting or diarrhoea, which could be a hint to metabolic alkalosis, were observed in the cats during this time. Moreover, the mean values for both groups regained normal levels within an additional week. Alterations in the blood chloride concentrations in the acute phase of FIV infection have to date not been published.

6.3.2.2.3.2 Blood Phosphorus Levels

The cats from both groups indicated increased phosphorus levels in blood during the entire duration of the experiment. This can be expected in young, growing animals. Moreover, increased phosphorus levels can be due to delayed serum separation after blood collections.

Significantly lower blood phosphorus levels were measured in the treated group during the treatment period and until week 1 post-challenge. As with many other parameters, slight divergences were already measured for this parameter before the onset of the treatment, rendering interpretation of this observation difficult. The increased values were still comprised in the normal range and therefore lacked clinical relevance.

6.3.3 Evaluation of Viral Infection

In order to test the efficacy of prophylactic treatment using dSLIM™, the outcome of FIV challenge was closely monitored in all cats. No trace of virus in the treated cats after challenge infection would have indicated optimal prophylactic stimulation of the immune system and dSLIM™-mediated resistance to infection and disease. However, considering that this CpG-containing molecule had never before been

Discussion

administered to the domestic cat, we were aware that many variables in the procedure of the experiment could affect the outcome of FIV challenge, rendering chances of observing the ideal scheme of total protection against infection relatively low. In the foreseeing of the more probable advent of partial protection, precise understanding of viral kinetics subsequent to treatment with dSLIM™ appeared to be of great importance. Thus, we chose to evaluate several parameters of viral infection, enabling the differentiation of biological levels of protection:

- Assessment of proviral loads in the lymphocytes of the cats enabled to determine both occurrence and time point of the establishment of infection

- Measurement of viral loads in plasma and saliva provided indications on the potential of the established provirus to induce production and liberation of new virions

- Evaluation of the infectivity of the viral particles present in plasma allowed accurate estimation of the risk of viral transmission by the infected cat

Quantitative evaluation and follow-up of the evolution of these parameters separately permitted precise comparison of viral kinetics between the groups and enabled accurate interpretation of the immunological processes induced by treatment with dSLIM™ (see section 6.3.4), providing hints about strength and mechanisms of protection. The results obtained by the measurements of these parameters in the course of the study are discussed in the following sections.

6.3.3.1 FIV Proviral Loads in Whole Blood

Generally, FIV provirus could be detected by quantitative real-time PCR in lymphocytes from the cats of both groups as of week 1 post-challenge infection

Discussion

already. The measured mean loads increased rapidly to reach a plateau level at week 3, and then remained stable for the rest of the experiment. For 2 individuals of the dSLIM™-treated group however, provirus could not be detected until week 4 after FIV challenge. Measures were repeated separately, in order to confirm the observed absence of FIV DNA in the samples. This 3-week delay before establishment of infection in the 2 cats M1 and T3 indicates a short term antiviral effect of the treatment. Hypothetically, prophylactic administration of dSLIM™ induced a favourable immunological status in these cats at the time point of FIV challenge, capable of controlling viral replication in the early phase of infection (see also 6.3.4). Unfortunately however, the induced immune mechanism was insufficient to permanently prevent establishment of infection, as proviral loads were comparable to those of control cats and the virus could replicate unhindered as of week 4 post-infection (more details in chapter 6.3.3.2).

The innate immune response elicited by CpG ODNs is known to enhance the host's defence mechanisms for about 2 weeks [359], and the effect of dSLIM™ was possibly of too short duration. Moreover, challenge infection with the particularly virulent FIV-GL8 strain may have been too aggressive in relation to the potency of the induced immune mechanisms.

Success in delaying the establishment of FIV infection in 2 cats of the dSLIM™-treated group can nevertheless be interpreted as partial protection of these 2 individuals in our experiment.

6.3.3.2 FIV Viral Loads

6.3.3.2.1 FIV Viral Load in Plasma

After rapidly increasing until week 2 post-challenge, the FIV loads measured in plasma by quantitative real-time PCR diminished gradually until the end of the study in both groups, indicating less active release of viral particles by the infected peripheral blood cells over time. This finding may coïncide with an increase in cytotoxic CD8+ T lymphocytes commonly observed at this stage of FIV infection [46, 385]. However, this statement remains speculative, as both quantitative measurements and evaluation of the function of this cell population have not been carried out in this study.

No virus could repeatedly be detected in the plasma of the 2 cats M1 and T3 which remained provirus negative until week 4 post-infection (see also 6.3.3.1). As of this time point however, similar viral loads as measured in the control group could be detected in plasma of these cats, not only confirming establishment of infection, but also indicating effective production and liberation of new viral particles by the infected lymphocytes. These observations altogether point to the induction of immune mechanisms capable of suppressing viral dissemination in the early phase of infection, insufficient however, in conferring total protection. The immune processes involved in the partial resistance to FIV observed in the 2 cats M1 and T3 are discussed in chapter 6.3.4.

6.3.3.2.2 FIV Viral Load in Saliva

As biting is considered the main mode of FIV transmission between cats, it seemed relevant to evaluate the effect of treatment with dSLIM™ on the shedding of FIV in saliva. Throughout the experiment, FIV RNA was quantitatively measured in saliva samples in weekly intervals. For both groups, 2 peaks of viral secretion in saliva were observed, namely at weeks 5 and 9 post infection. Between these time points, no FIV RNA could be detected in the saliva of any individual. Surprisingly, during the observed peaks, secretion of FIV was not only measured in more individuals from the dSLIM™-treated group, but the concerned animals also shed higher amounts of virus. With p-values of 0.09 for week 5 and 0.065 for week 9, these findings were relatively close to statistical significance. Altogether, these results remain rather difficult to interpret. Probably, a longer observation period would have enabled clearer understanding of the meaning and relevance of these peaks in viral secretion in saliva. Moreover, as little is known to date about the kinetics of FIV secretion in saliva, shorter intervals and study of various biological and behavioural factors would have been necessary to more precisely define shedding patterns and possible relation of the findings to the treatment with dSLIM™. An earlier study described

Discussion

continuous segregation of FIV in salivary gland tissue as of week 1 post-challenge infection, yet without obvious relation between the isolation rate from saliva and either clinical stage of disease or level of neutralizing antibodies in plasma [157]. Secretion of FIV in saliva may thus be correlated to triggers such as the occurrence of stressful situations or the act of biting. Such assumptions remain however purely hypothetical and require more detailed study.

Finally, our experiments indicate presence of virus in saliva, but not its infectivity. Isolation and subsequent quantitative measurements of infectious virus in saliva, in a similar manner as carried out in this study for the determination of infectious viral loads in plasma (see 6.3.3.3), would provide more accurate information on the odds of viral transmission at a given time point, and could be foreseen in the preparation of future studies.

6.3.3.3 Isolation of Virus from Plasma

Preseeded PBMCs isolated from a spf cat were weekly inoculated with the plasma of the cats enrolled in the study. The aim of this experiment was to test whether prophylactic treatment of the cats with dSLIM ™ affected the overall infectiosity of the viral particles present in plasma, i.e. their capacity of disseminating infection within the host by infecting new lymphocytes. This technique was preferred to others previously described using CRFK [386], MYA-1 [387], MBM [28], and Fet J [61] target cell lines because PBMCs closest reflect *in vivo* mechanisms. It should be mentioned that isolation of virus may be hampered by FIV neutralizing antibodies and cytokine activity present in the plasma used as substrate. As these parameters may vary over time and between individuals, this fact should be kept in mind when interpreting the results obtained with such an experiment.

Presence of virus in supernatants was determined by real time RT-PCR after 4 weeks of culture, as this amount of time ensures liberation of FIV by infected PBMCs *in vitro*. In order to certify that they reflected the presence of newly produced virus,

Discussion

results were compared quantitatively to real time RT-PCR measurements of a control consisting of infectious viral stock added to medium without cells, and held under same culture conditions.

For cost and time purposes, the experiment was carried out over 6 weeks, namely between weeks 2 and 8 after challenge infection. This short period of time seemed nevertheless sufficient, as it covers the acute phase of FIV infection with the particularly virulent GL8 strain used in this experiment. Infectious virus could be isolated from the samples obtained in the second week post-infection already in cats from both groups. By weeks 4 and 5 after challenge infection, production of infectious virus was detected in all cats from both groups, and in all but 1 individual from the dSLIM™-treated group at week 7 post-infection. Also, higher quantities of virus were generally measured for these time points, in comparison to weeks 2, 3 and 8 post-infection. Although the experiment was not carried out for week 6 post-challenge, the latter results seem to indicate a peak in infectious virus production between weeks 4, 5 and eventually 6 after experimental infection with FIV-GL8.

Higher mean amounts of infectious virus were detected in a greater number of individuals of the control group at both the second and third weeks after challenge. It could thus be speculated that treatment with dSLIM™ slightly delayed effective production of infectious virus in the cats. Such findings indicate a successful modification of the immunological status of the cats subsequent to treatment; the characterization of immune mechanisms carried out throughout this study can unfortunately only partially confirm such a hypothesis (see section 6.3.4). Somewhat significantly higher infectious viral loads were observed at week 8 after challenge infection in the treated group. The reasons for this finding remain unclear. Sample measurements in following weeks would have probably been necessary for a thorough interpretation of this result.

No infectious virus could be isolated until week 4 post-challenge from the 2 cats M1 and T3, which remained negative for proviral and viral loads during this period

Discussion

of time (see 6.3.3.2). Importantly, several control animals, which were positive with real-time PCR for both provirus and virus, also did not produce infectious virus until the fourth week post-infection. Presence of provirus or of virus in plasma thus did not always correlate with production of infectious virus. Unfortunately however, we could not significantly demonstrate suppression of infectious virus production by treatment with dSLIM™. Absence of infectious virus in the plasma of the 2 cats M1 and T3 nevertheless confirms their state of partial protection against FIV infection until week 4 post-challenge.

6.3.4 Immunological Measurements

Characterization of the immune response induced by the treatment with dSLIM™ was foreseen to enable both a precise evaluation of the *in vivo* immunomodulatory potential of this molecule in the domestic cat, and analysis of the background to the observed alterations in viral kinetics after FIV challenge.

The differentiation of naïve T cells in the course of an immune reaction to CD4+ Th1 cells or Th2 cells determines the network of defence mechanisms which is used by the organism to combat against infection. Manipulation of the innate immune system allows to influence the direction of this differenciation and this concept is today generally seen as feasible approach to help the body mount optimal responses against a very broad spectrum of pathogens [388, 389]. Promotion of Th1 immune responses is highly desired in the setting of viral diseases, because the cytokines produced by the Th1-differentiated CD4+ T cells enhance cellular defence mechanisms and suppress Th2 deviations, which rather induce humoral immunity. Th1 cells are known to produce high amounts of Il-12, IFN-γ and TNF-α, whereas Th2 cells mainly produce IL-4, IL-10 and IL-13.

Retroviral infections such as HIV, SIV and FIV naturally induce an early cellular immune response in the host, which reacts to viral proteins with a CTL response. This Th1-biased mechanism is unfortunately unsuccessful in inhibiting viral replication

Discussion

and dissemination. With progression of disease, chronic changes to the immune system appear, of which gradual increase in specific antibodies and decline in Th1 cell activities. This Th1 to Th2 orientation switch in active immune responses involves critical changes in the cytokine balance and has been described as potential influencial factor for the contraction of AIDS [390]. Moreover, Th2 immune responses have been repeatedly shown to either fail in protecting cats from an FIV challenge infection [391], or not to correlate with observed vaccine-induced protection [392]. The importance of supporting the early cellular immune responses in attempts to combat retroviral infections is thus widely accepted. In this way, prophylactic treatment of domestic cats with a potent CpG-containing molecule was intended to stimulate those components of the innate immune system which could emphasize and possibly maintain the early Th1 deviation of the immune mechanisms engendered by FIV challenge infection.

For a thorough interpretation of the viral kinetics observed in both groups during the present study, it seemed imperative to compare the balance between Th1 and Th2 immune reactions in treated and non-treated cats. Thus, we focused our immunological measurements on typical components of both Th1 and Th2 immune deviations. Antibody production, eosinophil granulocyte counts, as well as expression levels of IL-10 were analyzed in order to characterize the extent of a Th2 deviation. Detection of IL-12 p40 subunit mRNA levels was foreseen to typify a Th1-deviated immune response. Further possibilities to evaluate cellular immune responses include determination of specific CTL and NK cell counts along with analysis of their effector mechanisms. These parameters would have enabled a more precise illustration of the immune status of the cats during treatment and after FIV infection.

Through the determination of anti-FIV TM antibody titres with ELISA and the accomplishment of two separate cytokine experiments, we expected to show the Th1 effects of dSLIM™ *in vivo* in the domestic cat model and to demonstrate positive consequences on the immunological outcome of FIV challenge infection subsequent to administration of this molecule.

Discussion

6.3.4.1 Anti-TM ELISA

Weekly measurements of antibodies to FIV TM protein by ELISA were foreseen to compare the time point of seroconversion as well as the antibody titres in both groups throughout the experiment. In all cats of our study, seroconversion occurred by week 3 post-challenge. No significant differences were thereby observed between both groups. At several time points during the experiment, the individuals of the treated group indicated significanty higher antibody titres when compared to those of the control group. These findings were rather surprising, as humoral responses represent effective Th2 deviations, and treatment with dSLIM™ was foreseen to favor cellular immune mechanisms. The observed prolonged resistance to FIV infection in the 2 individuals from the treated group appeared to be nonetheless attributable to enhanced cellular immune responses, as these cats produced comparably low levels of antibodies until the fourth week post-challenge. NK cell and CTL cytotoxicity assays would have given more precise information on the nature of the immune mechanisms present in these cats and may be considered for future experiments.

In both groups, two clearly defined peaks of antibody production were observed at weeks 5 and 7 post-challenge. The mean titres seemed to stabilize towards the end of the experiment; analysis of this parameter at further time points would however be required to determine the presence of more peaks, and to enable their correct interpretation.

6.3.4.2 Cytokine Measurements

Measurements of cytokine expression in whole blood, as well as determination of the responsiveness to stimulation of isolated PBMCs from all cats allowed evaluation of both the systemic immune environment induced by dSLIM™ treatment and its effects on the course of subsequent FIV infection. Real-time RT-PCR techniques for the measurement of gene expression allowed the accurate determination of mRNA levels of the target genes Il-12 p40 and IL-10. In order to avoid experimental

Discussion

variations in the amount of RNA used in each real-time RT-PCR as well as eventual batch-to-batch variations in PCR reagents, coincident measurement of GAPDH, a catalytic enzyme produced by a so-called «housekeeping» gene, was used for the normalization of target gene expression data. An inherent assumption in the use of housekeeping genes is that their expression is ubiquitous and remains constant in the cells or tissues under investigation, regardless of age, gender or pathological alterations. Although the «house-keeping» status of GAPDH is relatively controversial, measurement of the expression of this gene remains to date the most commonly used method to standardize the analysis of expression of other cytokines [375, 376, 393].

6.3.4.2.1 Cytokine Expression in Whole Blood

Although great attention was attributed to the precision of the measurements of IL-10 and IL-12 p40 expressions in whole blood of the cats, it remained difficult to ensure the use, for TNA extractions prior to RT-PCR analysis of an amount of blood containing the same amount of cells for each cat. Thus, the measured divergences in GAPDH mRNA levels were most likely a result of unequal samples rather than of individual expression variations. As a result, comparative analysis regarding GAPDH expression for different individuals or between different time points gives little valuable information. Nevertheless, the graphical representation of GAPDH mRNA levels in this study hints that both dSLIM™ treatment and FIV infection had little or no effect on GAPDH expression, emphasizing the «housekeeping» state of the GAPDH gene. Moreover, the use of the TNA obtained from the extractions accomplished with the whole blood samples for the determination of all 3 parameters (GAPDH, IL-12 p40, IL-10), enabled to calculate the GAPDH: cytokine ratio and thus to feasibly standardize the results from the individual cats.

The expression of IL-10, a typical Th2 cytokine, could not be measured during the treatment period for both groups. In treated and non-treated cats, FIV challenge infection induced a rapid increase in IL-10 levels, which reflect the previously

Discussion

described development of Th2-deviated immune responses after infection with immunosuppressive retroviruses. However, the treated group presented lower mean IL-10 expression levels after challenge infection, indicating an expected Th2-suppressive effect of dSLIM™.

Disappointingly, very similar levels of IL-12 p40 subunit mRNA were measured in both groups during the treatment period. Moreover, rather unexpectedly, the IL-12 p40 expression levels of the treated group remained relatively unchanged after challenge, whereas the control group indicated a significant increase in mean expression levels of this cytokine. The presence of an early cellular immune response, as expected in the acute phase of infection, is most likely responsible for the observed IL-12 expression in the non-treated cats. However, as various experiments with dSLIM™ have shown potent induction of a Th1 environment *in vitro* and *in vivo* in different species, an insufficient duration of treatment or a suboptimal administration protocol of dSLIM™ could possibly be the reason for the apparent lack of IL-12 stimulation by the treatment. Moreover, as IL-12 is a typical Th1 cytokine, it seems unlikely that these results are a consequence of a suboptimal choice of target cytokine for these measurements.

6.3.4.2.2 Stimulation of Cytokine Expression *in vitro*

In order to assess to which extent PBMCs from treated cats can be more or less effectively stimulated to express certain cytokines, as well as to evaluate the effect of infection on their responsiveness to stimulation, various *in vitro* analyses were carried out at two strategic time points during the experiment, namely at week 0, before FIV challenge infection of the cats, and at week 8 post-challenge. Thereby, isolated PBMCs from each cat were either left unstimulated, or separately stimulated with Con A or LPS. These substances are known for their mitogenic potentials on T lymphocytes, and both have previously been shown to enhance the production of Th1 and Th2 cytokines *in vitro* [394]. Levels of GAPDH, IL-10 and IL-12 p40 subunit mRNA present in the isolated cells were measured by RT-PCR. This

Discussion

experiment was designed with the intention to confirm the results obtained by the measurements of these cytokines in whole blood, and to demonstrate a predisposition of lymphocytes from dSLIM™-treated cats to produce cytokines favouring Th1 or cellular immune mechanisms.

The graphics representing GAPDH levels appeared very similar for both time points. However, the columns for week 8 seemed to be generally shifted toward a lower level in comparison to those of week 0. Probably, by mistake, more cells had been isolated for the experiments on week 0 than for those on week 8. The higher GAPDH levels measured after Con A stimulation, at both weeks, is most likely due to proliferation of the cells between stimulation and harvesting time points. As a reminder, cell counts were only determined at the time point of isolation, and not after stimulation. Taking this hypothesis into consideration, GAPDH expression was most likely not influenced by stimulation. Moreover, FIV infection did not affect basal GAPDH mRNA levels in PBMCs and these infected cells could not be stimulated to increased production of this enzyme. Altogether, the well-known stability of GAPDH within the same individual and cell type cannot be questioned through these results.

In all cats, IL-10 could not be detected at week 0 in unstimulated PBMCs, indicating absence of a basal expression level of this cytokine. This observation confirms the measurements carried out for IL-10 in whole blood (see 6.3.4.2.1). Interestingly, stimulation of the PBMCs isolated from the control group at this time point, by both ConA and LPS, increased IL-10 liberation considerably. This was however not the case for the PBMCs isolated from the treated cats, as they could not significantly be stimulated to produce IL-10. Thus, as initially expected, it seems that the treatment with dSLIM™ suppressed expression of this Th2 cytokine. Surprisingly however, 8 weeks after FIV infection, known to induce in the host the progressive development of a Th2-deviated immune response, isolated PBMCs from the control cats were less, and PBMCs from treated cats more responsive to stimulation, when it came to IL-10 production. Cells isolated from the dSLIM™-treated cats were thereby

Discussion

particularly sensitive to stimulation with LPS. Generally, IL-10 expression by the PBMCs of both groups seemed more effective with Con A before and with LPS after FIV challenge. Partially similar observations have been formerly reported as responses of lymphocytes from infected cats were shown to less consistently respond to stimulation with Con A than cells from non-infected cats [59].

In accordance with the measurements accomplished in whole blood, a basal production of IL-12 p40 mRNA could be detected before FIV challenge in both groups. Significantly higher expression of this cytokine was observed in the treated group at week 0, supporting the hypothesis that administration of dSLIM™ to the cats in our experiment rapidly favoured the mounting of a Th1-oriented immune response. IL-12 p40 production by the isolated PBMCs could generally be stimulated slightly by Con A and considerably by LPS; disappointingly, PBMCs from the individuals of both groups thereby reacted similarly. As noted in the measurements completed in whole blood, IL-12 p40 levels detected in PBMCs post-infection were higher than at week 0 for both groups. Moreover, when compared to results obtained at week 0, PBMCs from the control group were significantly more susceptible to stimulation with LPS, whereas PBMCs from the treated group produced significantly less IL-12 p40 subsequent to the same stimulation at week 8 post-infection. These findings indicate that although treatment with dSLIM™ seems to have boosted early cellular defence mechanisms, the observed immunomodulatory effect lasted about 4 weeks in duration. Additional experiments during the acute phase of infection, at time points between weeks 0 and 8 post-challenge would most likely reveal valuable information in this respect.

Altogether, we could demonstrate a Th1-deviating immune effect subsequent to the 5-day administration of dSLIM™ to the cats. Indeed, before challenge infection, the PBMCs isolated from the treated cats not only produced significantly higher amounts of IL-12 than those from the control cats, but could not be stimulated to express IL-10. However, 8 weeks after experimental infection with FIV, the situation seemed to be somewhat inversed: The isolated lymphocytes from the

Discussion

dSLIM™-treated cats displayed a higher tendency to express IL-10, and the levels of IL-12 p40 detected in these individuals were similar to those measured in the control group. These observations contradict the facts published on cytokine responses to infection with FIV and remain difficult to explain.

6.4 Conclusion and Future Perspectives

In an era of permanent emergence of new health-threatening viral diseases which sporadically enter the human population from animal reservoirs, such as the severe acute respiratory syndrome (SARS) and avian influenza (avian flu), the development of novel strategies to diminish risks of pandemics is under great pressure. Although vaccination already commonly confers long term protection to a large variety of familiar infectious agents, the development of an effective, safe vaccine requires an enormous amount of time, allowing yet uncharacterized viruses to disseminate and lead to considerable damage. With respect to emerging viral pathogens, manipulation of the innate immune system has gained, in the last 10 years, incredible popularity as alternative to elicitation of specific immunity. Indeed, innate immunity not only initiates immediate reaction to a wide range of pathogens, but greatly supports the subsequent development of specific immune mechanisms. Moreover, the organism's first line of defence is known to possess the fantastic potential to instigate the production of powerful antiviral substances. Research groups worldwide are concentrating on elaborating the recent idea of inducing innate immune responses as prophylactic or therapeutic measures in the setting of infectious diseases. The availability of an appropriate outbred small animal model for such research purposes is therefore currently highly desirable.

The present work in is line with the scientific trend of this decade. We demonstrated that prophylactic stimulation of the innate immune system with a CpG-containing molecule is able to induce partial resistance against FIV infection. For the first time, the immunomodulatory potential of dSLIM™, a specifically constructed molecule exhibiting several CpG motifs, was evaluated *in vivo* in the domestic cat. Clinically

Discussion

very well tolerated, dSLIM™ induced only slight haematological alterations, namely transient increase in absolute neutrophil and monocyte counts. The partial protection observed in 2 cats from the dSLIM™-treated group was uttered by a 3-week delay in detection of both proviral and viral loads in blood. Additionally, no infectious virus could be isolated from the PBMCs of these individuals during this lapse of time. The virus was thus hindered in its establishment in the host for several weeks after challenge infection. These observations could be linked to suppressed anti-FIV antibody titres measured in these individuals in the acute phase of infection. Moreover, comparatively higher mean levels of IL-12 at the time point of challenge and lower mean IL-10 expression levels shortly after challenge infection were detected in the treated group. Altogether these findings emphasize the role of Th1-deviated immune mechanisms in the partial resistance against FIV infection observed in these 2 cats. As NK cells and CTL represent the main cell populations directly responsible for cellular immune responses, evaluation of their effector functions with NK cytotoxicity assays or detection of cytokines such as perforine and granzyme B would enable, in future experiments, to confirm and further characterize the immune processes involved in this protective mechanism. The evaluation of various IgG subclasses would also hint the presence of either Th1 or Th2 immune deviations. Such differentiation is however to date not possible due to the unavailability of tests for these feline antibodies on the market.

The complex network of feline innate immunity remains to date under-explored. Prophylactic stimulation of innate immune mechanisms with stand-alone agents is not only a very recent inspiration in medical research, but represents a true novelty in experiments concerning the domestic cat. Also, the immunomodulatory effects of dSLIM™ on the feline model had never before been investigated. As a consequence, this study was mainly based on hypothetical extrapolations from knowledge acquired through published experiments regarding other species and/or types of synthetic ODN. Many critical parameters thus most likely greatly affected the outcome of the present work. In this way, an *in vitro* optimization of dSLIM™ on feline immune cells, as well as a series of pre-experimental *in vivo* administration tests would help

Discussion

revise important factors such as viral challenge and injection protocols for future trials.

The promising results obtained despite the inevitable accumulation of such variables in our study adds up to several other factors favouring the use of a feline model for research on modulation of the innate immune system. As inbreeding and other detention conditions seem to have influenced their innate immune responses over time, laboratory animals like mice or rabbits somewhat deviate from ideal models for experiments concerning innate immunity. The domestic cat is an outbred species moreover affected by a variety of viral infections, such as FIV, FHV and FCoV which closely resemble in their biological properties those affecting humans or other species. Finally, host-virus interactions acquired throughout evolution render induction of antiviral resistance particularly challenging in the cat, thus increasing relevance of promising results for the human population. Collectively, these facts emphasize the feasibility to extend knowledge on the feline model as basis for further investigations concerning modulation of innate immunity. Our study suggests that non-specific prophylactic manipulation of the cat's early immune mechanisms holds the potential to induce resistance to a challenge viral infection. These findings open the way to future experiments which could change the face of medical science.

7. References

1. Miyazawa, T., et al., *Preliminary comparisons of the biological properties of two strains of feline immunodeficiency virus (FIV) isolated in Japan with FIV Petaluma strain isolated in the United States.* Arch Virol, 1989. 108(1-2): p. 59-68.

2. Talbott, R.L., et al., *Nucleotide sequence and genomic organization of feline immunodeficiency virus.* Proc Natl Acad Sci U S A, 1989. 86(15): p. 5743-7.

3. Sparger, E.E., et al., *Regulation of gene expression directed by the long terminal repeat of the feline immunodeficiency virus.* Virology, 1992. 187(1): p. 165-77.

4. Kemler, I., I. Azmi, and E.M. Poeschla, *The critical role of proximal gag sequences in feline immunodeficiency virus genome encapsidation.* Virology, 2004. 327(1): p. 111-20.

5. Tomonaga, K., et al., *Comparison of the Rev transactivation of feline immunodeficiency virus in feline and non-feline cell lines.* J Vet Med Sci, 1994. 56(1): p. 199-201.

6. Lockridge, K.M., et al., *Protective immunity against feline immunodeficiency virus induced by inoculation with vif-deleted proviral DNA.* Virology, 2000. 273(1): p. 67-79.

7. de Parseval, A. and J.H. Elder, *Demonstration that orf2 encodes the feline immunodeficiency virus transactivating (Tat) protein and characterization of a unique gene product with partial rev activity.* J Virol, 1999. 73(1): p. 608-17.

8. Chatterji, U., A. de Parseval, and J.H. Elder, *Feline immunodeficiency virus OrfA is distinct from other lentivirus transactivators.* J Virol, 2002. 76(19): p. 9624-34.

9. Gemeniano, M.C., E.T. Sawai, and E.E. Sparger, *Feline immunodeficiency virus Orf-A localizes to the nucleus and induces cell cycle arrest.* Virology, 2004. 325(2): p. 167-74.

10. Hosie, M.J., et al., *A monoclonal antibody which blocks infection with feline immunodeficiency virus identifies a possible non-CD4 receptor.* J Virol, 1993. 67(3): p. 1667-71.

11. de Parseval, A., et al., *Blocking of feline immunodeficiency virus infection by a monoclonal antibody to CD9 is via inhibition of virus release rather than interference with receptor binding.* J Virol, 1997. 71(8): p. 5742-9.

12. Richardson, J., et al., *Shared usage of the chemokine receptor CXCR4 by primary and laboratory-*

References

adapted strains of feline immunodeficiency virus. J Virol, 1999. 73(5) : p. 3661-71.

13. Willett, B.J., et al., *The second extracellular loop of CXCR4 determines its function as a receptor for feline immunodeficiency virus.* J Virol, 1998. 72(8): p. 6475-81.

14. Endo, Y., et al., *Inhibitory effect of stromal cell derived factor-1 on the replication of divergent strains of feline immunodeficiency virus in a feline T-lymphoid cell line.* Vet Immunol Immunopathol, 2000. 74(3-4): p. 303-14.

15. Egberink, H.F., et al., *Bicyclams, selective antagonists of the human chemokine receptor CXCR4, potently inhibit feline immunodeficiency virus replication.* J Virol, 1999. 73(8): p. 6346-52.

16. Lerner, D.L. and J.H. Elder, *Expanded host cell tropism and cytopathic properties of feline immunodeficiency virus strain PPR subsequent to passage through interleukin-2-independent T cells.* J Virol, 2000. 74(4): p. 1854-63.

17. Shimojima, M., et al., *Use of CD134 as a primary receptor by the feline immunodeficiency virus.* Science, 2004. 303(5661): p. 1192-5.

18. Verschoor, E.J., et al., *A single mutation within the V3 envelope neutralization domain of feline immunodeficiency virus determines its tropism for CRFK cells.* J Virol, 1995. 69(8) : p. 4752-7.

19. Johnston, J.B. and C. Power, *Feline immunodeficiency virus xenoinfection: the role of chemokine receptors and envelope diversity.* J Virol, 2002. 76(8): p. 3626-36.

20. Giannecchini, S., et al., *The membrane-proximal tryptophan-rich region in the transmembrane glycoprotein ectodomain of feline immunodeficiency virus is important for cell entry.* Virology, 2004. 320(1): p. 156-66.

21. Brown, W.C., et al., *Feline immunodeficiency virus infects both CD4+ and CD8+ T lymphocytes.* J Virol, 1991. 65(6): p. 3359-64.

22. Dean, G.A., et al., *Proviral burden and infection kinetics of feline immunodeficiency virus in lymphocyte subsets of blood and lymph node.* J Virol, 1996. 70(8): p. 5165-9.

23. Brunner, D. and N.C. Pedersen, *Infection of peritoneal macrophages in vitro and in vivo with feline immunodeficiency virus.* J Virol, 1989. 63(12): p. 5483-8.

24. Dow, S.W., C.K. Mathiason, and E.A. Hoover, *In vivo monocyte tropism of pathogenic feline immunodeficiency viruses.* J Virol, 1999. 73(8): p. 6852-61.

25. Dow, S.W., M.L. Poss, and E.A. Hoover, *Feline immunodeficiency virus: a neurotropic lentivirus.* J Acquir Immune Defic Syndr, 1990. 3(7): p. 658-68.

26. Martin, J.P., et al., *Evidence of feline immunodeficiency virus replication in cultured Kupffer cells.* Aids, 1995. 9(5): p. 447-53.

References

27. Lerner, D.L., et al., *FIV infection of IL-2-dependent and -independent feline lymphocyte lines: host cells range distinctions and specific cytokine upregulation.* Vet Immunol Immunopathol, 1998. 65(2-4): p. 277-97.

28. Matteucci, D., et al., *The feline lymphoid cell line MBM and its use for feline immunodeficiency virus isolation and quantitation.* Vet Immunol Immunopathol, 1995. 46(1-2): p. 71-82.

29. Ikeda, Y., et al., *Feline immunodeficiency virus can infect a human cell line (MOLT-4) but establishes a state of latency in the cells.* J Gen Virol, 1996. 77 (Pt 8): p. 1623-30.

30. Johnston, J. and C. Power, *Productive infection of human peripheral blood mononuclear cells by feline immunodeficiency virus: implications for vector development.* J Virol, 1999. 73(3): p. 2491-8.

31. Willett, B.J., et al., *Shared usage of the chemokine receptor CXCR4 by the feline and human immunodeficiency viruses.* J Virol, 1997. 71(9): p. 6407-15.

32. Whitwam, T., M. Peretz, and E. Poeschla, *Identification of a central DNA flap in feline immunodeficiency virus.* J Virol, 2001. 75(19): p. 9407-14.

33. Yamamoto, J.K., et al., *Pathogenesis of experimentally induced feline immunodeficiency virus infection in cats.* Am J Vet Res, 1988. 49(8): p. 1246-58.

34. Jordan, H.L., et al., *Feline immunodeficiency virus is shed in semen from experimentally and naturally infected cats.* AIDS Res Hum Retroviruses, 1998. 14(12): p. 1087-92.

35. Jordan, H.L., et al., *Transmission of feline immunodeficiency virus in domestic cats via artificial insemination.* J Virol, 1996. 70(11): p. 8224-8.

36. Wasmoen, T., et al., *Transmission of feline immunodeficiency virus from infected queens to kittens.* Vet Immunol Immunopathol, 1992. 35(1-2): p. 83-93.

37. Sellon, R.K., et al., *Feline immunodeficiency virus can be experimentally transmitted via milk during acute maternal infection.* J Virol, 1994. 68(5): p. 3380-5.

38. O'Neil, L.L., M.J. Burkhard, and E.A. Hoover, *Frequent perinatal transmission of feline immunodeficiency virus by chronically infected cats.* J Virol, 1996. 70(5): p. 2894-901.

39. Obert, L.A. and E.A. Hoover, *Feline immunodeficiency virus clade C mucosal transmission and disease courses.* AIDS Res Hum Retroviruses, 2000. 16(7): p. 677-88.

40. Bishop, S.A., et al., *Vaginal and rectal infection of cats with feline immunodeficiency virus.* Vet Microbiol, 1996. 51(3-4): p. 217-27.

41. Torten, M., et al., *Progressive immune dysfunction in cats experimentally infected with feline immunodeficiency virus.* J Virol, 1991. 65(5): p. 2225-30.

42. Hohdatsu, T., et al., *Ability of CD8+ T cell anti-feline immunodeficiency virus (FIV) activity*

References

and FIV proviral DNA load in mononuclear cells in FIV-infected cats. J Vet Med Sci, 2005. 67(1): p. 129-31.

43. Diehl, L.J., et al., *Plasma viral RNA load predicts disease progression in accelerated feline immunodeficiency virus infection.* J Virol, 1996. 70(4): p. 2503-7.

44. Guiot, A.L., D. Rigal, and G. Chappuis, *Spontaneous programmed cell death (PCD) process of lymphocytes of FIV-infected cats: cellular targets and modulation.* Vet Immunol Immunopathol, 1997. 58(2): p. 93-106.

45. Holznagel, E., et al., *The role of in vitro-induced lymphocyte apoptosis in feline immunodeficiency virus infection: correlation with different markers of disease progression.* J Virol, 1998. 72(11): p. 9025-33.

46. Willett, B.J., et al., *Infection with feline immunodeficiency virus is followed by the rapid expansion of a CD8+ lymphocyte subset.* Immunology, 1993. 78(1): p. 1-6.

47. Beatty, J.A., et al., *A longitudinal study of feline immunodeficiency virus-specific cytotoxic T lymphocytes in experimentally infected cats, using antigen-specific induction.* J Virol, 1996. 70(9): p. 6199-206.

48. Flynn, J.N., et al., *Involvement of cytolytic and non-cytolytic T cells in the control of feline immunodeficiency virus infection.* Vet Immunol Immunopathol, 2002. 85(3-4): p. 159-70.

49. Hohdatsu, T., M. Okubo, and H. Koyama, *Feline CD8+ T cell non-cytolytic anti-feline immunodeficiency virus activity mediated by a soluble factor(s).* J Gen Virol, 1998. 79 (Pt 11): p. 2729-35.

50. Hohdatsu, T., et al., *Studies on feline CD8+ T cell non-cytolytic anti-feline immunodeficiency virus (FIV) activity.* Arch Virol, 2000. 145(12): p. 2525-38.

51. Gebhard, D.H., et al., *Progressive expansion of an L-selectin-negative CD8 cell with anti-feline immunodeficiency virus (FIV) suppressor function in the circulation of FIV-infected cats.* J Infect Dis, 1999. 180(5): p. 1503-13.

52. Paillot, R., et al., *Toward a detailed characterization of feline immunodeficiency virus-specific T cell immune responses and mediated immune disorders.* Vet Immunol Immunopathol, 2005. 106(1-2): p. 1-14.

53. Tompkins, M.B., et al., *Feline immunodeficiency virus infection is characterized by B7+CTLA4+ T cell apoptosis.* J Infect Dis, 2002. 185(8): p. 1077-93.

54. Bull, M.E., et al., *Spontaneous T cell apoptosis in feline immunodeficiency virus (FIV)-infected cats is inhibited by IL2 and anti-B7.1 antibodies.* Vet Immunol Immunopathol, 2004. 99(1-2): p. 25-37.

55. Vahlenkamp, T.W., M.B. Tompkins, and W.A. Tompkins, *Feline immunodeficiency virus*

References

infection phenotypically and functionally activates immunosuppressive CD4+CD25+ T regulatory cells. J Immunol, 2004. 172(8): p. 4752-61.

56. Joshi, A., et al., *Preferential replication of FIV in activated CD4(+)CD25(+)T cells independent of cellular proliferation.* Virology, 2004. 321(2): p. 307-22.

57. Burkhard, M.J. and G.A. Dean, *Transmission and immunopathogenesis of FIV in cats as a model for HIV.* Curr HIV Res, 2003. 1(1): p. 15-29.

58. Dean, G.A. and N.C. Pedersen, *Cytokine response in multiple lymphoid tissues during the primary phase of feline immunodeficiency virus infection.* J Virol, 1998. 72(12): p. 9436-40.

59. Lawrence, C.E., et al., *Cytokine production by cats infected with feline immunodeficiency virus: a longitudinal study.* Immunology, 1995. 85(4): p. 568-74.

60. Kraus, L.A., et al., *Relationship between tumor necrosis factor alpha and feline immunodeficiency virus expressions.* J Virol, 1996. 70(1): p. 566-9.

61. Tanabe, T. and J.K. Yamamoto, *Feline immunodeficiency virus lacks sensitivity to the antiviral activity of feline IFN-gamma.* J Interferon Cytokine Res, 2001. 21(12): p. 1039-46.

62. Mizuno, T., et al., *TNF-alpha-induced cell death in feline immunodeficiency virus-infected cells is mediated by the caspase cascade.* Virology, 2001. 287(2): p. 446-55.

63. Flynn, J.N., et al., *Polyclonal B-cell activation in cats infected with feline immunodeficiency virus.* Immunology, 1994. 81(4): p. 626-30.

64. Levy, J.K., et al., *Elevated interleukin-10-to-interleukin-12 ratio in feline immunodeficiency virus-infected cats predicts loss of type 1 immunity to Toxoplasma gondii.* J Infect Dis, 1998. 178(2): p. 503-11.

65. Dean, G.A., J.A. Bernales, and N.C. Pedersen, *Effect of feline immunodeficiency virus on cytokine response to Listeria monocytogenes in vivo.* Vet Immunol Immunopathol, 1998. 65(2-4): p. 125-38.

66. Egberink, H.F., et al., *Humoral immune response to feline immunodeficiency virus in cats with experimentally induced and naturally acquired infections.* Am J Vet Res, 1992. 53(7): p. 1133-8.

67. Siebelink, K.H., et al., *Two different mutations in the envelope protein of feline immunodeficiency virus allow the virus to escape from neutralization by feline serum antibodies.* Vet Immunol Immunopathol, 1995. 46(1-2): p. 51-9.

68. Bendinelli, M., et al., *During readaptation in vivo, a tissue culture-adapted strain of feline immunodeficiency virus reverts to broad neutralization resistance at different times in individual hosts but through changes at the same position of the surface glycoprotein.* J Virol, 2001. 75(10): p. 4584-93.

69. Inoshima, Y., et al., *Persistence of high virus neutralizing antibody titers in cats experimentally*

References

infected with feline immunodeficiency virus. J Vet Med Sci, 1996. 58(9): p. 925-7.

70. Inoshima, Y., et al., *Cross virus neutralizing antibodies against feline immunodeficiency virus genotypes A, B, C, D and E.* Arch Virol, 1998. 143(1): p. 157-62.

71. Bachmann, M.H., et al., *Genetic diversity of feline immunodeficiency virus: dual infection, recombination, and distinct evolutionary rates among envelope sequence clades.* J Virol, 1997. 71(6): p. 4241-53.

72. Sodora, D.L., et al., *Identification of three feline immunodeficiency virus (FIV) env gene subtypes and comparison of the FIV and human immunodeficiency virus type 1 evolutionary patterns.* J Virol, 1994. 68(4): p. 2230-8.

73. Kakinuma, S., et al., *Nucleotide sequence of feline immunodeficiency virus: classification of Japanese isolates into two subtypes which are distinct from non-Japanese subtypes.* J Virol, 1995. 69(6): p. 3639-46.

74. Pecoraro, M.R., et al., *Genetic diversity of Argentine isolates of feline immunodeficiency virus.* J Gen Virol, 1996. 77 (Pt 9): p. 2031-5.

75. Kyaw-Tanner, M.T. and W.F. Robinson, *Quasispecies and naturally occurring superinfection in feline immunodeficiency virus infection.* Arch Virol, 1996. 141(9): p. 1703-13.

76. Motokawa, K., et al., *Mutations in feline immunodeficiency (FIV) virus envelope gene V3-V5 regions in FIV-infected cats.* Vet Microbiol, 2005. 106(1-2): p. 33-40.

77. Okada, S., et al., *Superinfection of cats with feline immunodeficiency virus subtypes A and B.* AIDS Res Hum Retroviruses, 1994. 10(12): p. 1739-46.

78. de Monte, M., et al., *A multivariate statistical analysis to follow the course of disease after infection of cats with different strains of the feline immunodeficiency virus (FIV).* J Virol Methods, 2002. 103(2): p. 157-70.

79. Olmsted, R.A., et al., *Worldwide prevalence of lentivirus infection in wild feline species: epidemiologic and phylogenetic aspects.* J Virol, 1992. 66(10): p. 6008-18.

80. Nishimura, Y., et al., *Interspecies transmission of feline immunodeficiency virus from the domestic cat to the Tsushima cat (Felis bengalensis euptilura) in the wild.* J Virol, 1999. 73(9): p. 7916-21.

81. Biek, R., et al., *Epidemiology, genetic diversity, and evolution of endemic feline immunodeficiency virus in a population of wild cougars.* J Virol, 2003. 77(17): p. 9578-89.

82. Brown, E.W., et al., *A lion lentivirus related to feline immunodeficiency virus: epidemiologic and phylogenetic aspects.* J Virol, 1994. 68(9): p. 5953-68.

83. Barr, M.C., et al., *Isolation of a highly cytopathic lentivirus from a nondomestic cat.* J Virol, 1995.

References

69(11): p. 7371-4.

84. Smirnova, N., et al., *Feline lentiviruses demonstrate differences in receptor repertoire and envelope structural elements.* Virology, 2005. 342(1): p. 60-76.

85. VandeWoude, S., S.J. O'Brien, and E.A. Hoover, *Infectivity of lion and puma lentiviruses for domestic cats.* J Gen Virol, 1997. 78 (Pt 4): p. 795-800.

86. VandeWoude, S., C.L. Hageman, and E.A. Hoover, *Domestic cats infected with lion or puma lentivirus develop anti-feline immunodeficiency virus immune responses.* J Acquir Immune Defic Syndr, 2003. 34(1): p. 20-31.

87. Johnston, J.B., et al., *Xenoinfection of nonhuman primates by feline immunodeficiency virus.* Curr Biol, 2001. 11(14): p. 1109-13.

88. Browning, M.T., et al., *Primate and feline lentivirus vector RNA packaging and propagation by heterologous lentivirus virions.* J Virol, 2001. 75(11): p. 5129-40.

89. Butera, S.T., et al., *Survey of veterinary conference attendees for evidence of zoonotic infection by feline retroviruses.* J Am Vet Med Assoc, 2000. 217(10): p. 1475-9.

90. Kanzaki, L.I. and D.J. Looney, *Feline immunodeficiency virus: a concise review.* Front Biosci, 2004. 9: p. 370-7.

91. Lutz, H., et al., *[Feline immunodeficiency virus in Switzerland: clinical aspects and epidemiology in comparison with feline leukemia virus and coronaviruses].* Schweiz Arch Tierheilkd, 1990. 132(5): p. 217-25.

92. Ueland, K. and H. Lutz, *Prevalence of feline leukemia virus and antibodies to feline immunodeficiency virus in cats in Norway.* Zentralbl Veterinarmed B, 1992. 39(1): p. 53-8.

93. Moraillon, A., *Feline immunodepressive retrovirus infections in France.* Vet Rec, 1990. 126(3): p. 68-9.

94. Bennett, M., et al., *Prevalence of antibody to feline immunodeficiency virus in some cat populations.* Vet Rec, 1989. 124(15): p. 397-8.

95. Hosie, M.J., C. Robertson, and O. Jarrett, *Prevalence of feline leukaemia virus and antibodies to feline immunodeficiency virus in cats in the United Kingdom.* Vet Rec, 1989. 125(11): p. 293-7.

96. Gruffydd-Jones, T.J., et al., *Serological evidence of feline immunodeficiency virus infection in UK cats from 1975-76.* Vet Rec, 1988. 123(22): p. 569-70.

97. Bandecchi, P., et al., *Prevalence of feline immunodeficiency virus and other retroviral infections in sick cats in Italy.* Vet Immunol Immunopathol, 1992. 31(3-4): p. 337-45.

98. Peri, E.V., et al., *Seroepidemiological and clinical survey of feline immunodeficiency virus infection*

References

in northern Italy. Vet Immunol Immunopathol, 1994. 40(4): p. 285-97.

99. Hartmann, K. and K. Hinze, *[Epidemiology and clinical aspects of FIV infection in Bavaria].* Tierarztl Prax, 1991. 19(5): p. 545-51.

100. Arjona, A., et al., *Seroepidemiological survey of infection by feline leukemia virus and immunodeficiency virus in Madrid and correlation with some clinical aspects.* J Clin Microbiol, 2000. 38(9): p. 3448-9.

101. Knotek, Z., et al., *Epidemiology of feline leukaemia and feline immunodeficiency virus infections in the Czech Republic.* Zentralbl Veterinarmed B, 1999. 46(10): p. 665-71.

102. Yilmaz, H., A. Ilgaz, and D.A. Harbour, *Prevalence of FIV and FeLV infections in cats in Istanbul.* J Feline Med Surg, 2000. 2(1): p. 69-70.

103. Grindem, C.B., et al., *Seroepidemiologic survey of feline immunodeficiency virus infection in cats of Wake County, North Carolina.* J Am Vet Med Assoc, 1989. 194(2): p. 226-8.

104. Yamamoto, J.K., et al., *Epidemiologic and clinical aspects of feline immunodeficiency virus infection in cats from the continental United States and Canada and possible mode of transmission.* J Am Vet Med Assoc, 1989. 194(2): p. 213-20.

105. Maruyama, S., et al., *Seroprevalence of Bartonella henselae, Toxoplasma gondii, FIV and FeLV infections in domestic cats in Japan.* Microbiol Immunol, 2003. 47(2): p. 147-53.

106. Lin, J.A., et al., *Seroepidemiological survey of feline retrovirus infections in cats in Taiwan in 1993 and 1994.* J Vet Med Sci, 1995. 57(1): p. 161-3.

107. Nakamura, K., et al., *Contrastive prevalence of feline retrovirus infections between northern and southern Vietnam.* J Vet Med Sci, 2000. 62(8): p. 921-3.

108. Malik, R., et al., *Prevalences of feline leukaemia virus and feline immunodeficiency virus infections in cats in Sydney.* Aust Vet J, 1997. 75(5): p. 323-7.

109. Muirden, A., *Prevalence of feline leukaemia virus and antibodies to feline immunodeficiency virus and feline coronavirus in stray cats sent to an RSPCA hospital.* Vet Rec, 2002. 150(20): p. 621-5.

110. Swinney, G.R., et al., *Feline t-lymphotropic virus (FTLV) (feline immunodeficiency virus infection) in cats in New Zealand.* N Z Vet J, 1989. 37(1): p. 41-3.

111. Pedersen, N.C., et al., *Virulence differences between two field isolates of feline immunodeficiency virus (FIV-APetaluma and FIV-CPGammar) in young adult specific pathogen free cats.* Vet Immunol Immunopathol, 2001. 79(1-2): p. 53-67.

112. Ishida, T. and I. Tomoda, *Clinical staging of feline immunodeficiency virus infection.* Nippon Juigaku Zasshi, 1990. 52(3): p. 645-8.

113. Pedersen, N.C., et al., *Feline immunodeficiency virus infection.* Vet Immunol Immunopathol,

1989. 21(1): p. 111-29.

114. del Fierro, G.M., et al., *Quantification of lymphadenopathy in experimentally induced feline immunodeficiency virus infection in domestic cats.* Vet Immunol Immunopathol, 1995. 46(1-2): p. 3-12.

115. Lappin, M.R., *Opportunistic infections associated with retroviral infections in cats.* Semin Vet Med Surg (Small Anim), 1995. 10(4): p. 244-50.

116. Weaver, C.C., et al., *Placental immunopathology and pregnancy failure in the FIV-infected cat.* Placenta, 2005. 26(2-3): p. 138-47.

117. Podell, M., et al., *AIDS-associated encephalopathy with experimental feline immunodeficiency virus infection.* J Acquir Immune Defic Syndr, 1993. 6(7): p. 758-71.

118. Poli, A., et al., *Circulating immune complexes and analysis of renal immune deposits in feline immunodeficiency virus-infected cats.* Clin Exp Immunol, 1995. 101(2): p. 254-8.

119. Barsanti, J.A., et al., *Relationship of lower urinary tract signs to seropositivity for feline immunodeficiency virus in cats.* J Vet Intern Med, 1996. 10(1): p. 34-8.

120. Poli, A., et al., *Malignant lymphoma associated with experimentally induced feline immunodeficiency virus infection.* J Comp Pathol, 1994. 110(4): p. 319-28.

121. Callanan, J.J., et al., *Histologic classification and immunophenotype of lymphosarcomas in cats with naturally and experimentally acquired feline immunodeficiency virus infections.* Vet Pathol, 1996. 33(3): p. 264-72.

122. Davidson, M.G., et al., *Feline immunodeficiency virus predisposes cats to acute generalized toxoplasmosis.* Am J Pathol, 1993. 143(5): p. 1486-97.

123. Lappin, M.R., et al., *Effect of feline immunodeficiency virus infection on Toxoplasma gondii-specific humoral and cell-mediated immune responses of cats with serologic evidence of toxoplasmosis.* J Vet Intern Med, 1993. 7(2): p. 95-100.

124. Cohen, N.D., et al., *Epizootiologic association between feline immunodeficiency virus infection and feline leukemia virus seropositivity.* J Am Vet Med Assoc, 1990. 197(2): p. 220-5.

125. Dua, N., et al., *An experimental study of primary feline immunodeficiency virus infection in cats and a historical comparison to acute simian and human immunodeficiency virus diseases.* Vet Immunol Immunopathol, 1994. 43(4): p. 337-55.

126. Shelton, G.H., et al., *Hematologic manifestations of feline immunodeficiency virus infection.* Blood, 1990. 76(6): p. 1104-9.

127. Hofmann-Lehmann, R., et al., *Parameters of disease progression in long-term experimental feline*

References

retrovirus (feline immunodeficiency virus and feline leukemia virus) infections: hematology, clinical chemistry, and lymphocyte subsets. Clin Diagn Lab Immunol, 1997. 4(1): p. 33-42.

128. Goto, Y., et al., *Association of plasma viral RNA load with prognosis in cats naturally infected with feline immunodeficiency virus.* J Virol, 2002. 76(19): p. 10079-83.

129. Ishida, T., et al., *Feline immunodeficiency virus infection in cats of Japan.* J Am Vet Med Assoc, 1989. 194(2): p. 221-5.

130. Shelton, G.H., et al., *Feline immunodeficiency virus and feline leukemia virus infections and their relationships to lymphoid malignancies in cats: a retrospective study (1968-1988).* J Acquir Immune Defic Syndr, 1990. 3(6): p. 623-30.

131. Tenorio, A.P., et al., *Chronic oral infections of cats and their relationship to persistent oral carriage of feline calici-, immunodeficiency, or leukemia viruses.* Vet Immunol Immunopathol, 1991. 29(1-2): p. 1-14.

132. Knowles, J.O., et al., *Prevalence of feline calicivirus, feline leukaemia virus and antibodies to FIV in cats with chronic stomatitis.* Vet Rec, 1989. 124(13): p. 336-8.

133. Dawson, S., et al., *Effect of primary-stage feline immunodeficiency virus infection on subsequent feline calicivirus vaccination and challenge in cats.* Aids, 1991. 5(6): p. 747-50.

134. Reubel, G.H., et al., *Interaction of acute feline herpesvirus-1 and chronic feline immunodeficiency virus infections in experimentally infected specific pathogen free cats.* Vet Immunol Immunopathol, 1992. 35(1-2): p. 95-119.

135. Egberink, H.F., et al., *Papillomavirus associated skin lesions in a cat seropositive for feline immunodeficiency virus.* Vet Microbiol, 1992. 31(2-3): p. 117-25.

136. Brown, A., M. Bennett, and C.J. Gaskell, *Fatal poxvirus infection in association with FIV infection.* Vet Rec, 1989. 124(1): p. 19-20.

137. Pedersen, N.C., et al., *Feline leukemia virus infection as a potentiating cofactor for the primary and secondary stages of experimentally induced feline immunodeficiency virus infection.* J Virol, 1990. 64(2): p. 598-606.

138. Mancianti, F., et al., *Mycological findings in feline immunodeficiency virus-infected cats.* J Med Vet Mycol, 1992. 30(3): p. 257-9.

139. Witt, C.J., et al., *Epidemiologic observations on feline immunodeficiency virus and Toxoplasma gondii coinfection in cats in Baltimore, Md.* J Am Vet Med Assoc, 1989. 194(2): p. 229-33.

140. Lappin, M.R., et al., *Effect of primary phase feline immunodeficiency virus infection on cats with chronic toxoplasmosis.* Vet Immunol Immunopathol, 1992. 35(1-2): p. 121-31.

References

141. Mtambo, M.M., et al., *Cryptosporidium infection in cats: prevalence of infection in domestic and feral cats in the Glasgow area.* Vet Rec, 1991. 129(23): p. 502-4.

142. Hopper, C.D., et al., *Clinical and laboratory findings in cats infected with feline immunodeficiency virus.* Vet Rec, 1989. 125(13): p. 341-6.

143. Ferrer, L., et al., *Cryptococcosis in two cats seropositive for feline immunodeficiency virus.* Vet Rec, 1992. 131(17): p. 393-4.

144. Dandekar, S., et al., *Detection of feline immunodeficiency virus (FIV) nucleic acids in FIV-seronegative cats.* J Virol, 1992. 66(7): p. 4040-9.

145. Hartmann, K., et al., *[Diagnosis of FIV infection].* Tierarztl Prax, 1994. 22(3): p. 268-72.

146. Lutz, H., et al., *Specificity assessment of feline T-lymphotropic lentivirus serology.* Zentralbl Veterinarmed B, 1988. 35(10): p. 773-8.

147. Bennett, M., et al., *Diagnosis of FIV infection.* Vet Rec, 1989. 124(19): p. 520-1.

148. Calandrella, M., et al., *Densitometric analysis of Western blot assays for feline immunodeficiency virus antibodies.* Vet Immunol Immunopathol, 2001. 79(3-4): p. 261-71.

149. Reid, G., et al., *Immunodiagnosis of feline immunodeficiency virus infection using recombinant viral p17 and p24.* Aids, 1991. 5(12): p. 1477-83.

150. Fevereiro, M., C. Roneker, and F. de Noronha, *Antibody response to reverse transcriptase in cats infected with feline immunodeficiency virus.* Viral Immunol, 1991. 4(4): p. 225-35.

151. Furuya, T., et al., *Detection of anti-gag antibodies of feline immunodeficiency virus in cat sera by enzyme-linked immunosorbent assay.* Arch Virol, 1992. 124(3-4): p. 355-61.

152. Calzolari, M., et al., *Serological diagnosis of feline immunodeficiency virus infection using recombinant transmembrane glycoprotein.* Vet Immunol Immunopathol, 1995. 46(1-2): p. 83-92.

153. Kashiwase, H., et al., *Characterization of one monoclonal antibody against feline immunodeficiency virus p24 and its application to antigen capture ELISA.* J Virol Methods, 1997. 68(2): p. 183-92.

154. Guiot, A.L., et al., *Development of a simple, rapid and accurate in vitro whole blood technique for the detection and semi-quantification of FIV cellular viremia.* Vet Microbiol, 1995. 47(3-4): p. 331-42.

155. Hohdatsu, T., et al., *Detection of feline immunodeficiency proviral DNA in peripheral blood lymphocytes by the polymerase chain reaction.* Vet Microbiol, 1992. 30(2-3): p. 113-23.

156. Rimstad, E. and K. Ueland, *Detection of feline immunodeficiency virus by a nested polymerase chain reaction.* J Virol Methods, 1992. 36(3): p. 239-48.

References

157. Matteucci, D., et al., *Detection of feline immunodeficiency virus in saliva and plasma by cultivation and polymerase chain reaction.* J Clin Microbiol, 1993. 31(3): p. 494-501.

158. Inoshima, Y., et al., *Quantification of feline immunodeficiency virus (FIV) proviral DNA in peripheral blood mononuclear cells of cats infected with Japanese strains of FIV.* J Vet Med Sci, 1995. 57(3): p. 487-92.

159. Vahlenkamp, T.W., et al., *Competitive reverse transcription-polymerase chain reaction for quantitation of feline immunodeficiency virus.* J Virol Methods, 1995. 52(3): p. 335-46.

160. Leutenegger, C.M., et al., *Rapid feline immunodeficiency virus provirus quantitation by* , 1999. 78(1-2): p. 105-16.

161. Rogers, A.B., C.K. Mathiason, and E.A. Hoover, *Immunohistochemical localization of feline immunodeficiency virus using native species antibodies.* Am J Pathol, 2002. 161(4): p. 1143-51.

162. North, T.W., et al., *Direct comparisons of inhibitor sensitivities of reverse transcriptases from feline and human immunodeficiency viruses.* Antimicrob Agents Chemother, 1990. 34(8): p. 1505-7.

163. Meers, J., et al., *Feline immunodeficiency virus infection: plasma, but not peripheral blood mononuclear cell virus titer is influenced by zidovudine and cyclosporine.* Arch Virol, 1993. 132(1-2): p. 67-81.

164. Hart, S. and I. Nolte, *Long-term treatment of diseased, FIV-seropositive field cats with azidothymidine (AZT).* Zentralbl Veterinarmed A, 1995. 42(6): p. 397-409.

165. Arai, M., D.D. Earl, and J.K. Yamamoto, *Is AZT/3TC therapy effective against FIV infection or immunopathogenesis?* Vet Immunol Immunopathol, 2002. 85(3-4): p. 189-204.

166. Uckun, F.M., et al., *In vivo antiretroviral activity of stampidine in chronically feline immunodeficiency virus-infected cats.* Antimicrob Agents Chemother, 2003. 47(4): p. 1233-40.

167. Auwerx, J., et al., *Chimeric human immunodeficiency virus type 1 and feline immunodeficiency virus reverse transcriptases: role of the subunits in resistance/sensitivity to non-nucleoside reverse transcriptase inhibitors.* Mol Pharmacol, 2002. 61(2): p. 400-6.

168. Auwerx, J., et al., *Susceptibility of feline immunodeficiency virus/human immunodeficiency virus type 1 reverse transcriptase chimeras to non-nucleoside RT inhibitors.* Mol Pharmacol, 2004. 65(1): p. 244-51.

169. Lee, T., et al., *Analysis of the S3 and S3' subsite specificities of feline immunodeficiency virus (FIV) protease: development of a broad-based protease inhibitor efficacious against FIV, SIV, and HIV in vitro and ex vivo.* Proc Natl Acad Sci U S A, 1998. 95(3): p. 939-44.

170. de Rozieres, S., et al., *Assessment of FIV-C infection of cats as a function of treatment with the*

protease inhibitor, TL-3. Retrovirology, 2004. 1(1): p. 38.

171. Huitron-Resendiz, S., et al., *Resolution and prevention of feline immunodeficiency virus-induced neurological deficits by treatment with the protease inhibitor TL-3.* J Virol, 2004. 78(9): p. 4525-32.

172. Lombardi, S., et al., *Inhibition of feline immunodeficiency virus infection in vitro by envelope glycoprotein synthetic peptides.* Virology, 1996. 220(2): p. 274-84.

173. Giannecchini, S., et al., *Antiviral activity and conformational features of an octapeptide derived from the membrane-proximal ectodomain of the feline immunodeficiency virus transmembrane glycoprotein.* J Virol, 2003. 77(6): p. 3724-33.

174. Giannecchini, S., et al., *Feline immunodeficiency virus plasma load reduction by a retroinverso octapeptide reproducing the Trp-rich motif of the transmembrane glycoprotein.* Antivir Ther, 2005. 10(5): p. 671-80.

175. Riondato, F., et al., *Effects of interferon alpha (INF-alpha) therapy on peripheral blood lymphocyte subsets from FIV and FeLV naturally infected cats.* Vet Res Commun, 2003. 27 Suppl 1: p. 429-32.

176. de Mari, K., et al., *Therapeutic effects of recombinant feline interferon-omega on feline leukemia virus (FeLV)-infected and FeLV/feline immunodeficiency virus (FIV)-coinfected symptomatic cats.* J Vet Intern Med, 2004. 18(4): p. 477-82.

177. Phillips, K., et al., *FIV-infected cats respond to short-term rHuG-CSF treatment which results in anti-G-CSF neutralizing antibody production that inactivates drug activity.* Vet Immunol Immunopathol, 2005. 108(3-4): p. 357-71.

178. Barr, M.C., et al., *Exogenous glucocorticoids alter parameters of early feline immunodeficiency virus infection.* J Infect Dis, 2000. 181(2): p. 576-86.

179. Mortola, E., et al., *The use of two immunosuppressive drugs, cyclosporin A and tacrolimus, to inhibit virus replication and apoptosis in cells infected with feline immunodeficiency virus.* Vet Res Commun, 1998. 22(8): p. 553-63.

180. Leutenegger, C.M., et al., *Immunization of cats against feline immunodeficiency virus (FIV) infection by using minimalistic immunogenic defined gene expression vector vaccines expressing FIV gp140 alone or with feline interleukin-12 (IL-12), IL-16, or a CpG motif.* J Virol, 2000. 74(22): p. 10447-57.

181. Pu, R., et al., *Dual-subtype FIV vaccine protects cats against in vivo swarms of both homologous and heterologous subtype FIV isolates.* Aids, 2001. 15(10): p. 1225-37.

182. Hartmann, K., *Feline immunodeficiency virus infection: an overview.* Vet J, 1998. 155(2): p. 123-37.

References

183. Hohdatsu, T., et al., *Passive antibody protection of cats against feline immunodeficiency virus infection.* J Virol, 1993. 67(4): p. 2344-8.

184. Pu, R., et al., *Protection of neonatal kittens against feline immunodeficiency virus infection with passive maternal antiviral antibodies.* Aids, 1995. 9(3): p. 235-42.

185. Pu, R., M.C. Tellier, and J.K. Yamamoto, *Mechanism(s) of FIV vaccine protection.* Leukemia, 1997. 11 Suppl 3: p. 98-101.

186. Pu, R., et al., *MHC-restricted protection of cats against FIV infection by adoptive transfer of immune cells from FIV-vaccinated donors.* Cell Immunol, 1999. 198(1): p. 30-43.

187. Yamamoto, J.K., et al., *Experimental vaccine protection against feline immunodeficiency virus.* AIDS Res Hum Retroviruses, 1991. 7(11): p. 911-22.

188. Hosie, M.J., et al., *Protection against homologous but not heterologous challenge induced by inactivated feline immunodeficiency virus vaccines.* J Virol, 1995. 69(2): p. 1253-5.

189. Hosie, M.J., et al., *Vaccination with inactivated virus but not viral DNA reduces virus load following challenge with a heterologous and virulent isolate of feline immunodeficiency virus.* J Virol, 2000. 74(20): p. 9403-11.

190. Matteucci, D., et al., *AIDS vaccination studies using feline immunodeficiency virus as a model: immunisation with inactivated whole virus suppresses viraemia levels following intravaginal challenge with infected cells but not following intravenous challenge with cell-free virus.* Vaccine, 1999. 18(1-2): p. 119-30.

191. Verschoor, E.J., et al., *Vaccination against feline immunodeficiency virus using fixed infected cells.* Vet Immunol Immunopathol, 1995. 46(1-2): p. 139-49.

192. Yamamoto, J.K., et al., *Experimental vaccine protection against homologous and heterologous strains of feline immunodeficiency virus.* J Virol, 1993. 67(1): p. 601-5.

193. Matteucci, D., et al., *Vaccination protects against in vivo-grown feline immunodeficiency virus even in the absence of detectable neutralizing antibodies.* J Virol, 1996. 70(1): p. 617-22.

194. Giannecchini, S., et al., *AIDS vaccination studies using an ex vivo feline immunodeficiency virus model: failure to protect and possible enhancement of challenge infection by four cell-based vaccines prepared with autologous lymphoblasts.* J Virol, 2002. 76(14): p. 6882-92.

195. Hohdatsu, T., et al., *Effect of dual-subtype vaccine against feline immunodeficiency virus infection.* Vet Microbiol, 1997. 58(2-4): p. 155-65.

196. Huang, C., et al., *Efficacy and safety of a feline immunodeficiency virus vaccine.* Anim Health Res Rev, 2004. 5(2): p. 295-300.

References

197. Pu, R., et al., *Dual-subtype FIV vaccine (Fel-O-Vax FIV) protection against a heterologous subtype B FIV isolate.* J Feline Med Surg, 2005. 7(1): p. 65-70.

198. Kusuhara, H., et al., *Dual-subtype vaccine (Fel-O-Vax FIV) protects cats against contact challenge with heterologous subtype B FIV infected cats.* Vet Microbiol, 2005. 108(3-4): p. 155-65.

199. Matteucci, D., et al., *Studies of AIDS vaccination using an ex vivo feline immunodeficiency virus model: protection conferred by a fixed-cell vaccine against cell-free and cell-associated challenge differs in duration and is not easily boosted.* J Virol, 1997. 71(11): p. 8368-76.

200. Chiarantini, L., et al., *AIDS vaccination studies using an ex vivo feline immunodeficiency virus model: homologous erythrocytes as a delivery system for preferential immunization with putative protective antigens.* Clin Diagn Lab Immunol, 1998. 5(2): p. 235-41.

201. Matteucci, D., et al., *Immunogenicity of an anti-clade B feline immunodeficiency fixed-cell virus vaccine in field cats.* J Virol, 2000. 74(23): p. 10911-9.

202. Lutz, H., et al., *FIV vaccine studies. I. Immune response to recombinant FIV env gene products and outcome after challenge infection.* Vet Immunol Immunopathol, 1995. 46(1-2): p. 103-13.

203. Leutenegger, C.M., et al., *Partial protection by vaccination with recombinant feline immunodeficiency virus surface glycoproteins.* AIDS Res Hum Retroviruses, 1998. 14(3): p. 275-83.

204. Hosie, M.J., et al., *Suppression of virus burden by immunization with feline immunodeficiency virus Env protein.* Vaccine, 1996. 14(5): p. 405-11.

205. Coleman, J.K., et al., *HIV-1 p24 vaccine protects cats against feline immunodeficiency virus infection.* Aids, 2005. 19(14): p. 1457-66.

206. Flynn, J.N., et al., *Induction of feline immunodeficiency virus-specific cell-mediated and humoral immune responses following immunization with a multiple antigenic peptide from the envelope V3 domain.* Immunology, 1995. 85(2): p. 171-5.

207. Flynn, J.N., et al., *Vaccination with a feline immunodeficiency virus multiepitopic peptide induces cell-mediated and humoral immune responses in cats, but does not confer protection.* J Virol, 1997. 71(10): p. 7586-92.

208. Gonin, P., et al., *Immunization trial of cats with a replication-defective adenovirus type 5 expressing the ENV gene of feline immunodeficiency virus.* Vet Microbiol, 1995. 45(4): p. 393-401.

209. Verschoor, E.J., et al., *Evaluation of subunit vaccines against feline immunodeficiency virus infection.* Vaccine, 1996. 14(4): p. 285-9.

210. Burkhard, M.J., et al., *Evaluation of FIV protein-expressing VEE-replicon vaccine vectors in cats.* Vaccine, 2002. 21(3-4): p. 258-68.

211. Tellier, M.C., et al., *Efficacy evaluation of prime-boost protocol: canarypoxvirus-based feline*

References

immunodeficiency virus (FIV) vaccine and inactivated FIV-infected cell vaccine against heterologous FIV challenge in cats. Aids, 1998. 12(1): p. 11-8.

212. Osterhaus, A.D., et al., *Accelerated viremia in cats vaccinated with recombinant vaccinia virus expressing envelope glycoprotein of feline immunodeficiency virus.* AIDS Res Hum Retroviruses, 1996. 12(5): p. 437-41.

213. Hosie, M.J., et al., *DNA vaccination affords significant protection against feline immunodeficiency virus infection without inducing detectable antiviral antibodies.* J Virol, 1998. 72(9): p. 7310-9.

214. Dunham, S.P., et al., *Protection against feline immunodeficiency virus using replication defective proviral DNA vaccines with feline interleukin-12 and -18.* Vaccine, 2002. 20(11-12): p. 1483-96.

215. Pistello, M., et al., *Evaluation of feline immunodeficiency virus ORF-A mutants as candidate attenuated vaccine.* Virology, 2005. 332(2): p. 676-90.

216. Boretti, F.S., et al., *Protection against FIV challenge infection by genetic vaccination using minimalistic DNA constructs for FIV env gene and feline IL-12 expression.* Aids, 2000. 14(12): p. 1749-57.

217. Hosie, M.J., et al., *Enhancement after feline immunodeficiency virus vaccination.* Vet Immunol Immunopathol, 1992. 35(1-2): p. 191-7.

218. Karlas, J.A., et al., *Vaccination with experimental feline immunodeficiency virus vaccines, based on autologous infected cells, elicits enhancement of homologous challenge infection.* J Gen Virol, 1999. 80 (Pt 3): p. 761-5.

219. Siebelink, K.H., et al., *Enhancement of feline immunodeficiency virus infection after immunization with envelope glycoprotein subunit vaccines.* J Virol, 1995. 69(6): p. 3704-11.

220. Richardson, J., et al., *Enhancement of feline immunodeficiency virus (FIV) infection after DNA vaccination with the FIV envelope.* J Virol, 1997. 71(12): p. 9640-9.

221. Broche-Pierre, S., et al., *Evaluation of live feline immunodeficiency virus vaccines with modified antigenic properties.* J Gen Virol, 2005. 86(Pt 9): p. 2495-506.

222. Akira, S., K. Takeda, and T. Kaisho, *Toll-like receptors: critical proteins linking innate and acquired immunity.* Nat Immunol, 2001. 2(8): p. 675-80.

223. Janeway, C.A., Jr. and R. Medzhitov, *Innate immune recognition.* Annu Rev Immunol, 2002. 20: p. 197-216.

224. Beutler, B., et al., *How we detect microbes and respond to them: the Toll-like receptors and their transducers.* J Leukoc Biol, 2003. 74(4): p. 479-85.

225. Lemaitre, B., et al., *The dorsoventral regulatory gene cassette spatzle/Toll/cactus controls the potent*

References

antifungal response in Drosophila adults. Cell, 1996. 86(6): p. 973-83.

226. Imler, J.L. and J.A. Hoffmann, *Toll receptors in innate immunity.* Trends Cell Biol, 2001. 11(7): p. 304-11.

227. Slack, J.L., et al., *Identification of two major sites in the type I interleukin-1 receptor cytoplasmic region responsible for coupling to pro-inflammatory signaling pathways.* J Biol Chem, 2000. 275(7): p. 4670-8.

228. Ozinsky, A., et al., *Co-operative induction of pro-inflammatory signaling by Toll-like receptors.* J Endotoxin Res, 2000. 6(5): p. 393-6.

229. Dunne, A. and L.A. O'Neill, *The interleukin-1 receptor/Toll-like receptor superfamily: signal transduction during inflammation and host defense.* Sci STKE, 2003. 2003(171): p. re3.

230. Ahmad-Nejad, P., et al., *Bacterial CpG-DNA and lipopolysaccharides activate Toll-like receptors at distinct cellular compartments.* Eur J Immunol, 2002. 32(7): p. 1958-68.

231. Ulevitch, R.J., *Therapeutics targeting the innate immune system.* Nat Rev Immunol, 2004. 4(7): p. 512-20.

232. Takeda, K., T. Kaisho, and S. Akira, *Toll-like receptors.* Annu Rev Immunol, 2003. 21: p. 335-76.

233. Tabeta, K., et al., *Toll-like receptors 9 and 3 as essential components of innate immune defense against mouse cytomegalovirus infection.* Proc Natl Acad Sci U S A, 2004. 101(10): p. 3516-21.

234. Bird, A.P., *DNA methylation and the frequency of CpG in animal DNA.* Nucleic Acids Res, 1980. 8(7): p. 1499-504.

235. Karlin, S., W. Doerfler, and L.R. Cardon, *Why is CpG suppressed in the genomes of virtually all small eukaryotic viruses but not in those of large eukaryotic viruses?* J Virol, 1994. 68(5): p. 2889-97.

236. Sun, S., et al., *Type I interferon-mediated stimulation of T cells by CpG DNA.* J Exp Med, 1998. 188(12): p. 2335-42.

237. Wagner, H., *Bacterial CpG DNA activates immune cells to signal infectious danger.* Adv Immunol, 1999. 73: p. 329-68.

238. Hemmi, H., et al., *A Toll-like receptor recognizes bacterial DNA.* Nature, 2000. 408(6813): p. 740-5.

239. Chuang, T.H. and R.J. Ulevitch, *Cloning and characterization of a sub-family of human toll-like receptors: hTLR7, hTLR8 and hTLR9.* Eur Cytokine Netw, 2000. 11(3): p. 372-8.

240. Takeshita, F., et al., *Cutting edge: Role of Toll-like receptor 9 in CpG DNA-induced activation of human cells.* J Immunol, 2001. 167(7): p. 3555-8.

241. Bauer, S., et al., *Human TLR9 confers responsiveness to bacterial DNA via species-specific CpG*

References

motif recognition. Proc Natl Acad Sci U S A, 2001. 98(16): p. 9237-42.

242. Latz, E., et al., *Mechanisms of TLR9 activation.* J Endotoxin Res, 2004. 10(6): p. 406-12.

243. Hacker, H., et al., *CpG-DNA-specific activation of antigen-presenting cells requires stress kinase activity and is preceded by non-specific endocytosis and endosomal maturation.* Embo J, 1998. 17(21): p. 6230-40.

244. Rutz, M., et al., *Toll-like receptor 9 binds single-stranded CpG-DNA in a sequence- and pH-dependent manner.* Eur J Immunol, 2004. 34(9): p. 2541-50.

245. Barton, G.M., J.C. Kagan, and R. Medzhitov, *Intracellular localization of Toll-like receptor 9 prevents recognition of self DNA but facilitates access to viral DNA.* Nat Immunol, 2006. 7(1): p. 49-56.

246. Zhao, Q., et al., *Comparison of cellular binding and uptake of antisense phosphodiester, phosphorothioate, and mixed phosphorothioate and methylphosphonate oligonucleotides.* Antisense Res Dev, 1993. 3(1): p. 53-66.

247. Lee, S.W., et al., *Effects of a hexameric deoxyriboguanosine run conjugation into CpG oligodeoxynucleotides on their immunostimulatory potentials.* J Immunol, 2000. 165(7): p. 3631-9.

248. Bauer, S. and H. Wagner, *Bacterial CpG-DNA licenses TLR9.* Curr Top Microbiol Immunol, 2002. 270: p. 145-54.

249. Hacker, H., et al., *Immune cell activation by bacterial CpG-DNA through myeloid differentiation marker 88 and tumor necrosis factor receptor-associated factor (TRAF)6.* J Exp Med, 2000. 192(4): p. 595-600.

250. Gao, J.J., et al., *Regulation of gene expression in mouse macrophages stimulated with bacterial CpG-DNA and lipopolysaccharide.* J Leukoc Biol, 2002. 72(6): p. 1234-45.

251. Bast, R.C., Jr., et al., *BCG and cancer.* N Engl J Med, 1974. 290(26): p. 1458-69.

252. Yamamoto, S., et al., *In vitro augmentation of natural killer cell activity and production of interferon-alpha/beta and -gamma with deoxyribonucleic acid fraction from Mycobacterium bovis BCG.* Jpn J Cancer Res, 1988. 79(7): p. 866-73.

253. Kuramoto, E., et al., *Oligonucleotide sequences required for natural killer cell activation.* Jpn J Cancer Res, 1992. 83(11): p. 1128-31.

254. Yamamoto, S., et al., *DNA from bacteria, but not from vertebrates, induces interferons, activates natural killer cells and inhibits tumor growth.* Microbiol Immunol, 1992. 36(9): p. 983-97.

255. Messina, J.P., G.S. Gilkeson, and D.S. Pisetsky, *The influence of DNA structure on the in vitro stimulation of murine lymphocytes by natural and synthetic polynucleotide antigens.* Cell Immunol,

1993. 147(1): p. 148-57.

256. Krieg, A.M., et al., *CpG motifs in bacterial DNA trigger direct B-cell activation.* Nature, 1995. 374(6522): p. 546-9.

257. Hartmann, G. and A.M. Krieg, *Mechanism and function of a newly identified CpG DNA motif in human primary B cells.* J Immunol, 2000. 164(2): p. 944-53.

258. Hartmann, G., et al., *Delineation of a CpG phosphorothioate oligodeoxynucleotide for activating primate immune responses in vitro and in vivo.* J Immunol, 2000. 164(3): p. 1617-24.

259. Brown, W.C., et al., *DNA and a CpG oligonucleotide derived from Babesia bovis are mitogenic for bovine B cells.* Infect Immun, 1998. 66(11): p. 5423-32.

260. Rankin, R., et al., *CpG motif identification for veterinary and laboratory species demonstrates that sequence recognition is highly conserved.* Antisense Nucleic Acid Drug Dev, 2001. 11(5): p. 333-40.

261. Yi, A.K., et al., *Rapid immune activation by CpG motifs in bacterial DNA. Systemic induction of IL-6 transcription through an antioxidant-sensitive pathway.* J Immunol, 1996. 157(12): p. 5394-402.

262. Yi, A.K., et al., *CpG DNA rescue of murine B lymphoma cells from anti-IgM-induced growth arrest and programmed cell death is associated with increased expression of c-myc and bcl-xL.* J Immunol, 1996. 157(11): p. 4918-25.

263. Yi, A.K., et al., *CpG oligodeoxyribonucleotides rescue mature spleen B cells from spontaneous apoptosis and promote cell cycle entry.* J Immunol, 1998. 160(12): p. 5898-906.

264. Wang, Z., et al., *Unmethylated CpG motifs protect murine B lymphocytes against Fas-mediated apoptosis.* Cell Immunol, 1997. 180(2): p. 162-7.

265. Sparwasser, T., et al., *Bacterial DNA and immunostimulatory CpG oligonucleotides trigger maturation and activation of murine dendritic cells.* Eur J Immunol, 1998. 28(6): p. 2045-54.

266. Hartmann, G., G.J. Weiner, and A.M. Krieg, *CpG DNA: a potent signal for growth, activation, and maturation of human dendritic cells.* Proc Natl Acad Sci U S A, 1999. 96(16): p. 9305-10.

267. Kadowaki, N., et al., *Subsets of human dendritic cell precursors express different toll-like receptors and respond to different microbial antigens.* J Exp Med, 2001. 194(6): p. 863-9.

268. Krug, A., et al., *Toll-like receptor expression reveals CpG DNA as a unique microbial stimulus for plasmacytoid dendritic cells which synergizes with CD40 ligand to induce high amounts of IL-12.* Eur J Immunol, 2001. 31(10): p. 3026-37.

269. Osada, T., et al., *Peripheral blood dendritic cells, but not monocyte-derived dendritic cells, can augment human NK cell function.* Cell Immunol, 2001. 213(1): p. 14-23.

270. Ban, E., et al., *CpG motifs induce Langerhans cell migration in vivo.* Int Immunol, 2000. 12(6):

References

p. 737-45.

271. Baek, K.H., S.J. Ha, and Y.C. Sung, *A novel function of phosphorothioate oligodeoxynucleotides as chemoattractants for primary macrophages.* J Immunol, 2001. 167(5): p. 2847-54.

272. Lipford, G.B., et al., *Immunostimulatory DNA: sequence-dependent production of potentially harmful or useful cytokines.* Eur J Immunol, 1997. 27(12): p. 3420-6.

273. Shimada, S., O. Yano, and T. Tokunaga, *In vivo augmentation of natural killer cell activity with a deoxyribonucleic acid fraction of BCG.* Jpn J Cancer Res, 1986. 77(8): p. 808-16.

274. Yamamoto, S., et al., U*nique palindromic sequences in synthetic oligonucleotides are required to induce IFN [correction of INF] and augment IFN-mediated [correction of INF] natural killer activity.* J Immunol, 1992. 148(12): p. 4072-6.

275. Ballas, Z.K., W.L. Rasmussen, and A.M. Krieg, *Induction of NK activity in murine and human cells by CpG motifs in oligodeoxynucleotides and bacterial DNA.* J Immunol, 1996. 157(5): p. 1840-5.

276. Cowdery, J.S., et al., *Bacterial DNA induces NK cells to produce IFN-gamma in vivo and increases the toxicity of lipopolysaccharides.* J Immunol, 1996. 156(12): p. 4570-5.

277. Krug, A., et al., *Identification of CpG oligonucleotide sequences with high induction of IFN-alpha/beta in plasmacytoid dendritic cells.* Eur J Immunol, 2001. 31(7): p. 2154-63.

278. Marschner, A., et al., *CpG ODN enhance antigen-specific NKT cell activation via plasmacytoid dendritic cells.* Eur J Immunol, 2005. 35(8): p. 2347-57.

279. Marshall, J.D., et al., *Induction of interferon-gamma from natural killer cells by immunostimulatory CpG DNA is mediated through plasmacytoid-dendritic-cell-produced interferon-alpha and tumour necrosis factor-alpha.* Immunology, 2006. 117(1): p. 38-46.

280. Agrawal, S. and E.R. Kandimalla, *Medicinal chemistry and therapeutic potential of CpG DNA.* Trends Mol Med, 2002. 8(3): p. 114-21.

281. Pasare, C. and R. Medzhitov, *Toll pathway-dependent blockade of CD4+CD25+ T cell-mediated suppression by dendritic cells.* Science, 2003. 299(5609): p. 1033-6.

282. Weighardt, H., et al., *Increased resistance against acute polymicrobial sepsis in mice challenged with immunostimulatory CpG oligodeoxynucleotides is related to an enhanced innate effector cell response.* J Immunol, 2000. 165(8): p. 4537-43.

283. Klinman, D.M., et al., *CpG motifs present in bacteria DNA rapidly induce lymphocytes to secrete interleukin 6, interleukin 12, and interferon gamma.* Proc Natl Acad Sci U S A, 1996. 93(7): p. 2879-83.

284. Lipford, G.B., et al., *CpG-DNA-mediated transient lymphadenopathy is associated with a state of*

Th1 predisposition to antigen-driven responses. J Immunol, 2000. 165(3): p. 1228-35.

285. Kobayashi, H., et al., *Immunostimulatory DNA pre-priming: a novel approach for prolonged Th1-biased immunity.* Cell Immunol, 1999. 198(1): p. 69-75.

286. Liu, Y.J., *IPC: professional type 1 interferon-producing cells and plasmacytoid dendritic cell precursors.* Annu Rev Immunol, 2005. 23 : p. 275-306.

287. Santini, S.M., et al., *Type I interferon as a powerful adjuvant for monocyte-derived dendritic cell development and activity in vitro and in Hu-PBL-SCID mice.* J Exp Med, 2000. 191(10): p. 1777-88.

288. Poeck, H., et al., *Plasmacytoid dendritic cells, antigen, and CpG-C license human B cells for plasma cell differentiation and immunoglobulin production in the absence of T-cell help.* Blood, 2004. 103(8): p. 3058-64.

289. Agnello, D., et al., *Cytokines and transcription factors that regulate T helper cell differentiation: new players and new insights.* J Clin Immunol, 2003. 23(3): p. 147-61.

290. Verthelyi, D. and D.M. Klinman, *Immunoregulatory activity of CpG oligonucleotides in humans and nonhuman primates.* Clin Immunol, 2003. 109(1): p. 64-71.

291. Wernette, C.M., et al., *CpG oligodeoxynucleotides stimulate canine and feline immune cell proliferation.* Vet Immunol Immunopathol, 2002. 84(3-4): p. 223-36.

292. Sheehan, J.P. and H.C. Lan, *Phosphorothioate oligonucleotides inhibit the intrinsic tenase complex.* Blood, 1998. 92(5): p. 1617-25.

293. Henry, S.P., et al., *Complement activation is responsible for acute toxicities in rhesus monkeys treated with a phosphorothioate oligodeoxynucleotide.* Int Immunopharmacol, 2002. 2(12): p. 1657-66.

294. Heikenwalder, M., et al., *Lymphoid follicle destruction and immunosuppression after repeated CpG oligodeoxynucleotide administration.* Nat Med, 2004. 10(2): p. 187-92.

295. Brown, D.A., et al., *Effect of phosphorothioate modification of oligodeoxynucleotides on specific protein binding.* J Biol Chem, 1994. 269(43): p. 26801-5.

296. Verthelyi, D., et al., *Human peripheral blood cells differentially recognize and respond to two distinct CPG motifs.* J Immunol, 2001. 166(4): p. 2372-7.

297. Ito, S., et al., *CpG oligodeoxynucleotides improve the survival of pregnant and fetal mice following Listeria monocytogenes infection.* Infect Immun, 2004. 72(6): p. 3543-8.

298. Ito, S., et al., *CpG oligodeoxynucleotides enhance neonatal resistance to Listeria infection.* J Immunol, 2005. 174(2): p. 777-82.

299. Jahrsdorfer, B. and G.J. Weiner, *CpG oligodeoxynucleotides for immune stimulation in cancer*

References

immunotherapy. Curr Opin Investig Drugs, 2003. 4(6): p. 686-90.

300. Carpentier, A.F., G. Auf, and J.Y. Delattre, *CpG-oligonucleotides for cancer immunotherapy: review of the literature and potential applications in malignant glioma.* Front Biosci, 2003. 8: p. e115-27.

301. Baines, J. and E. Celis, *Immune-mediated tumor regression induced by CpG-containing oligodeoxynucleotides.* Clin Cancer Res, 2003. 9(7): p. 2693-700.

302. Heckelsmiller, K., et al., *Combined dendritic cell- and CpG oligonucleotide-based immune therapy cures large murine tumors that resist chemotherapy.* Eur J Immunol, 2002. 32(11): p. 3235-45.

303. Kawarada, Y., et al., *NK- and CD8(+) T cell-mediated eradication of established tumors by peritumoral injection of CpG-containing oligodeoxynucleotides.* J Immunol, 2001. 167(9): p. 5247-53.

304. Jahrsdorfer, B. and G.J. Weiner, *Immunostimulatory CpG oligodeoxynucleotides and antibody therapy of cancer.* Semin Oncol, 2003. 30(4): p. 476-82.

305. Weigel, B.J., et al., *CpG oligodeoxynucleotides potentiate the antitumor effects of chemotherapy or tumor resection in an orthotopic murine model of rhabdomyosarcoma.* Clin Cancer Res, 2003. 9(8): p. 3105-14.

306. Milas, L., et al., *CpG oligodeoxynucleotide enhances tumor response to radiation.* Cancer Res, 2004. 64(15): p. 5074-7.

307. Warren, T.L., C.E. Dahle, and G.J. Weiner, *CpG oligodeoxynucleotides enhance monoclonal antibody therapy of a murine lymphoma.* Clin Lymphoma, 2000. 1(1): p. 57-61.

308. Zwaveling, S., et al., *Established human papillomavirus type 16-expressing tumors are effectively eradicated following vaccination with long peptides.* J Immunol, 2002. 169(1): p. 350-8.

309. Miconnet, I., et al., *CpG are efficient adjuvants for specific CTL induction against tumor antigen-derived peptide.* J Immunol, 2002. 168(3): p. 1212-8.

310. Kim, T.Y., et al., *Both E7 and CpG-oligodeoxynucleotide are required for protective immunity against challenge with human papillomavirus 16 (E6/E7) immortalized tumor cells: involvement of CD4+ and CD8+ T cells in protection.* Cancer Res, 2002. 62(24): p. 7234-40.

311. Davila, E. and E. Celis, *Repeated administration of cytosine-phosphorothiolated guanine-containing oligonucleotides together with peptide/protein immunization results in enhanced CTL responses with anti-tumor activity.* J Immunol, 2000. 165(1): p. 539-47.

312. Uhlmann, E. and J. Vollmer, *Recent advances in the development of immunostimulatory oligonucleotides.* Curr Opin Drug Discov Devel, 2003. 6(2): p. 204-17.

313. Paul, S., *Technology evaluation: CpG-7909, Coley.* Curr Opin Mol Ther, 2003. 5(5): p. 553-9.

314. Friedberg, J.W., et al., *Combination immunotherapy with a CpG oligonucleotide (1018 ISS) and*

References

rituximab in patients with non-Hodgkin lymphoma: increased interferon-alpha/beta-inducible gene expression, without significant toxicity. Blood, 2005. 105(2): p. 489-95.

315. Krieg, A.M., *CpG motifs: the active ingredient in bacterial extracts?* Nat Med, 2003. 9(7): p. 831-5.

316. Pichardo, D.A., et al., *Cutaneous T-cell lymphoma: a paradigm for biological therapies.* Leuk Lymphoma, 2004. 45(9): p. 1755-65.

317. Cooper, C.L., et al., *CPG 7909, an immunostimulatory TLR9 agonist oligodeoxynucleotide, as adjuvant to Engerix-B HBV vaccine in healthy adults: a double-blind phase I/II study.* J Clin Immunol, 2004. 24(6): p. 693-701.

318. Siegrist, C.A., et al., *Co-administration of CpG oligonucleotides enhances the late affinity maturation process of human anti-hepatitis B vaccine response.* Vaccine, 2004. 23(5): p. 615-22.

319. Halperin, S.A., et al., *A phase I study of the safety and immunogenicity of recombinant hepatitis B surface antigen co-administered with an immunostimulatory phosphorothioate oligonucleotide adjuvant.* Vaccine, 2003. 21(19-20): p. 2461-7.

320. Schetter, C. and J. Vollmer, *Toll-like receptors involved in the response to microbial pathogens: development of agonists for toll-like receptor 9.* Curr Opin Drug Discov Devel, 2004. 7(2): p. 204-10.

321. Creticos, P.S. and L.M. Lichtenstein, *Progress in the development of new methods of immunotherapy: potential application of immunostimulatory DNA-conjugated to allergens for treatment of allergic respiratory conditions.* Arb Paul Ehrlich Inst Bundesamt Sera Impfstoffe Frankf A M, 2003(94): p. 304-12; discussion 312-3.

322. Vollmer, J., *Progress in drug development of immunostimulatory CpG oligodeoxynucleotide ligands for TLR9.* Expert Opin Biol Ther, 2005. 5(5): p. 673-82.

323. Kline, J.N., et al., *Modulation of airway inflammation by CpG oligodeoxynucleotides in a murine model of asthma.* J Immunol, 1998. 160(6): p. 2555-9.

324. Broide, D., et al., *Immunostimulatory DNA sequences inhibit IL-5, eosinophilic inflammation, and airway hyperresponsiveness in mice.* J Immunol, 1998. 161(12): p. 7054-62.

325. Sur, S., et al., *Long term prevention of allergic lung inflammation in a mouse model of asthma by CpG oligodeoxynucleotides.* J Immunol, 1999. 162(10): p. 6284-93.

326. Kline, J.N., et al., T*reatment of established asthma in a murine model using CpG oligodeoxynucleotides.* Am J Physiol Lung Cell Mol Physiol, 2002. 283(1): p. L170-9.

327. Jain, V.V., et al., *CpG-oligodeoxynucleotides inhibit airway remodeling in a murine model of chronic asthma.* J Allergy Clin Immunol, 2002. 110(6): p. 867-72.

328. Simons, F.E., et al., *Selective immune redirection in humans with ragweed allergy by injecting*

References

Amb a 1 linked to immunostimulatory DNA. J Allergy Clin Immunol, 2004. 113(6): p. 1144-51.

329. Tulic, M.K., et al., *Amb a 1-immunostimulatory oligodeoxynucleotide conjugate immunotherapy decreases the nasal inflammatory response.* J Allergy Clin Immunol, 2004. 113(2): p. 235-41.

330. Zimmermann, S., et al., *CpG oligodeoxynucleotides trigger protective and curative Th1 responses in lethal murine leishmaniasis.* J Immunol, 1998. 160(8): p. 3627-30.

331. Verthelyi, D., et al., *CpG oligodeoxynucleotides protect normal and SIV-infected macaques from Leishmania infection.* J Immunol, 2003. 170(9): p. 4717-23.

332. Elkins, K.L., et al., *Bacterial DNA containing CpG motifs stimulates lymphocyte-dependent protection of mice against lethal infection with intracellular bacteria.* J Immunol, 1999. 162(4): p. 2291-8.

333. Klinman, D.M., J. Conover, and C. Coban, *Repeated administration of synthetic oligodeoxynucleotides expressing CpG motifs provides long-term protection against bacterial infection.* Infect Immun, 1999. 67(11): p. 5658-63.

334. Babiuk, L.A., S. Gomis, and R. Hecker, *Molecular approaches to disease control.* Poult Sci, 2003. 82(6): p. 870-5.

335. Gomis, S., et al., *Protection of neonatal chicks against a lethal challenge of Escherichia coli using DNA containing cytosine-phosphodiester-guanine motifs.* Avian Dis, 2004. 48(4): p. 813-22.

336. He, H., et al., *In vitro activation of chicken leukocytes and in vivo protection against Salmonella enteritidis organ invasion and peritoneal S. enteritidis infection-induced mortality in neonatal chickens by immunostimulatory CpG oligodeoxynucleotide.* FEMS Immunol Med Microbiol, 2005. 43(1): p. 81-9.

337. Pyles, R.B., et al., *Use of immunostimulatory sequence-containing oligonucleotides as topical therapy for genital herpes simplex virus type 2 infection.* J Virol, 2002. 76(22): p. 11387-96.

338. Dong, L., et al., *An immunostimulatory oligodeoxynucleotide containing a cytidine-guanosine motif protects senescence-accelerated mice from lethal influenza virus by augmenting the T helper type 1 response.* J Gen Virol, 2003. 84(Pt 6): p. 1623-8.

339. Olbrich, A.R., et al., *Effective postexposure treatment of retrovirus-induced disease with immunostimulatory DNA containing CpG motifs.* J Virol, 2002. 76(22): p. 11397-404.

340. Olbrich, A.R., S. Schimmer, and U. Dittmer, *Preinfection treatment of resistant mice with CpG oligodeoxynucleotides renders them susceptible to friend retrovirus-induced leukemia.* J Virol, 2003. 77(19): p. 10658-62.

341. Schlaepfer, E., et al., *CpG oligodeoxynucleotides block human immunodeficiency virus type 1 replication in human lymphoid tissue infected ex vivo.* J Virol, 2004. 78(22): p. 12344-54.

References

342. Scheller, C., et al., *CpG oligodeoxynucleotides activate HIV replication in latently infected human T cells.* J Biol Chem, 2004. 279(21): p. 21897-902.

343. Gramzinski, R.A., et al., *Interleukin-12- and gamma interferon-dependent protection against malaria conferred by CpG oligodeoxynucleotide in mice.* Infect Immun, 2001. 69(3): p. 1643-9.

344. Deng, J.C., et al., *CpG oligodeoxynucleotides stimulate protective innate immunity against pulmonary Klebsiella infection.* J Immunol, 2004. 173(8): p. 5148-55.

345. Juffermans, N.P., et al., *CpG oligodeoxynucleotides enhance host defense during murine tuberculosis.* Infect Immun, 2002. 70(1): p. 147-52.

346. Rees, D.G., et al., *CpG-DNA protects against a lethal orthopoxvirus infection in a murine model.* Antiviral Res, 2005. 65(2): p. 87-95.

347. Reinis, M., J. Simova, and J. Bubenik, *Inhibitory effects of unmethylated CpG oligodeoxynucleotides on MHC class I-deficient and -proficient HPV16-associated tumours.* Int J Cancer, 2006. 118(7): p. 1836-42.

348. Hayashi, T., et al., *CpG oligodeoxynucleotides accelerate reovirus type 2-triggered insulitis in DBA/1 suckling mice.* Int J Exp Pathol, 2002. 83(5): p. 217-23.

349. Ito, S., J. Pedras-Vasconcelos, and D.M. Klinman, *CpG oligodeoxynucleotides increase the susceptibility of normal mice to infection by Candida albicans.* Infect Immun, 2005. 73(9): p. 6154-6.

350. Klinman, D.M., *Therapeutic applications of CpG-containing oligodeoxynucleotides.* Antisense Nucleic Acid Drug Dev, 1998. 8(2): p. 181-4.

351. Tighe, H., et al., *Conjugation of protein to immunostimulatory DNA results in a rapid, long-lasting and potent induction of cell-mediated and humoral immunity.* Eur J Immunol, 2000. 30(7): p. 1939-47.

352. Gursel, I., et al., *Sterically stabilized cationic liposomes improve the uptake and immunostimulatory activity of CpG oligonucleotides.* J Immunol, 2001. 167(6): p. 3324-8.

353. Moldoveanu, Z., et al., *CpG DNA, a novel immune enhancer for systemic and mucosal immunization with influenza virus.* Vaccine, 1998. 16(11-12): p. 1216-24.

354. Kovarik, J., et al., *CpG oligodeoxynucleotides can circumvent the Th2 polarization of neonatal responses to vaccines but may fail to fully redirect Th2 responses established by neonatal priming.* J Immunol, 1999. 162(3): p. 1611-7.

355. Oxenius, A., et al., *CpG-containing oligonucleotides are efficient adjuvants for induction of protective antiviral immune responses with T-cell peptide vaccines.* J Virol, 1999. 73(5): p. 4120-6.

356. Davis, H.L., et al., *CpG DNA is a potent enhancer of specific immunity in mice immunized with*

References

recombinant hepatitis B surface antigen. J Immunol, 1998. 160(2): p. 870-6.

357. Eastcott, J.W., et al., *Oligonucleotide containing CpG motifs enhances immune response to mucosally or systemically administered tetanus toxoid.* Vaccine, 2001. 19(13-14): p. 1636-42.

358. Prince, G.A., et al., *Immunoprotective activity and safety of a respiratory syncytial virus vaccine: mucosal delivery of fusion glycoprotein with a CpG oligodeoxynucleotide adjuvant.* J Virol, 2003. 77(24): p. 13156-60.

359. Klinman, D.M., et al., *Use of CpG oligodeoxynucleotides as immune adjuvants.* Immunol Rev, 2004. 199: p. 201-16.

360. Klinman, D.M., et al., *DNA vaccines: safety and efficacy issues.* Springer Semin Immunopathol, 1997. 19(2): p. 245-56.

361. Krieg, A.M., et al., *Sequence motifs in adenoviral DNA block immune activation by stimulatory CpG motifs.* Proc Natl Acad Sci U S A, 1998. 95(21): p. 12631-6.

362. Davis, H.L., *Use of CpG DNA for enhancing specific immune responses.* Curr Top Microbiol Immunol, 2000. 247: p. 171-83.

363. Gilkeson, G.S., et al., *Induction of immune-mediated glomerulonephritis in normal mice immunized with bacterial DNA.* Clin Immunol Immunopathol, 1993. 68(3): p. 283-92.

364. Gilkeson, G.S., A.M. Pippen, and D.S. Pisetsky, *Induction of cross-reactive anti-dsDNA antibodies in preautoimmune NZB/NZW mice by immunization with bacterial DNA.* J Clin Invest, 1995. 95(3): p. 1398-402.

365. Sparwasser, T., et al., *Macrophages sense pathogens via DNA motifs: induction of tumor necrosis factor-alpha-mediated shock.* Eur J Immunol, 1997. 27(7): p. 1671-9.

366. Verthelyi, D., et al., *CpG oligodeoxynucleotides as vaccine adjuvants in primates.* J Immunol, 2002. 168(4): p. 1659-63.

367. Livak, K.J., et al., *Oligonucleotides with fluorescent dyes at opposite ends provide a quenched probe system useful for detecting PCR product and nucleic acid hybridization.* PCR Methods Appl, 1995. 4(6): p. 357-62.

368. Chi, D.S. and N.S. Harris, *A simple method for the isolation of murine peripheral blood lymphocytes.* J Immunol Methods, 1978. 19(2-3): p. 169-72.

369. Klein, D., et al., *Influence of preassay and sequence variations on viral load determination by a multiplex real-time reverse transcriptase-polymerase chain reaction for feline immunodeficiency virus.* J Acquir Immune Defic Syndr, 2001. 26(1): p. 8-20.

370. Tandon, R., et al., *Quantitation of feline leukaemia virus viral and proviral loads by TaqMan*

real-time polymerase chain reaction. J Virol Methods, 2005. 130(1-2): p. 124-32.

371. Vogtlin, A., et al., *HSV-1-based amplicon particles are able to transduce cells of feline origin with genes encoding biologically functional feline IL-10 or IL-6.* Vet Microbiol, 2002. 86(1-2): p. 103-13.

372. Helps, C., et al., *Melting curve analysis of feline calicivirus isolates detected by real-time reverse transcription PCR.* J Virol Methods, 2002. 106(2): p. 241-4.

373. Gut, M., et al., *One-tube fluorogenic reverse transcription-polymerase chain reaction for the quantitation of feline coronaviruses.* J Virol Methods, 1999. 77(1): p. 37-46.

374. Wittig, B., et al., *Therapeutic vaccination against metastatic carcinoma by expression-modulated and immunomodified autologous tumor cells: a first clinical phase I/II trial.* Hum Gene Ther, 2001. 12(3): p. 267-78.

375. Leutenegger, C.M., et al., *Quantitative real-time PCR for the measurement of feline cytokine mRNA.* Vet Immunol Immunopathol, 1999. 71(3-4): p. 291-305.

376. Kipar, A., et al., *Cytokine mRNA levels in isolated feline monocytes.* Vet Immunol Immunopathol, 2001. 78(3-4): p. 305-15.

377. Der, S.D., et al., *Identification of genes differentially regulated by interferon alpha, beta, or gamma using oligonucleotide arrays.* Proc Natl Acad Sci U S A, 1998. 95(26): p. 15623-8.

378. Shpaer, E.G. and J.I. Mullins, *Selection against CpG dinucleotides in lentiviral genes: a possible role of methylation in regulation of viral expression.* Nucleic Acids Res, 1990. 18(19): p. 5793-7.

379. Schmidt, M., et al., *Cytokine and Ig-production by CG-containing sequences with phosphorodiester backbone and dumbbell-shape.* Allergy, 2006. 61(1): p. 56-63.

380. Kochling, J., et al., *Protection of mice against Philadelphia chromosome-positive acute immunomodulatory oligonucleotides.* Clin Cancer Res, 2003. 9(8): p. 3142-9.

381. Weihrauch, M.R., et al., *Phase I/II combined chemoimmunotherapy with carcinoembryonic antigen-derived HLA-A2-restricted CAP-1 peptide and irinotecan, 5-fluorouracil, and leucovorin in patients with primary metastatic colorectal cancer.* Clin Cancer Res, 2005. 11(16): p. 5993-6001.

382. Klinman, D.M., *Immunotherapeutic uses of CpG oligodeoxynucleotides.* Nat Rev Immunol, 2004. 4(4): p. 249-58.

383. Shelton, G.H. and M.L. Linenberger, *Hematologic abnormalities associated with retroviral infections in the cat.* Semin Vet Med Surg (Small Anim), 1995. 10(4): p. 220-33.

384. Barlough, J.E., et al., *Acquired immune dysfunction in cats with experimentally induced feline immunodeficiency virus infection: comparison of short-term and long-term infections.* J Acquir Immune Defic Syndr, 1991. 4(3): p. 219-27.

References

385. Ackley, C.D., et al., *Immunologic abnormalities in pathogen-free cats experimentally infected with feline immunodeficiency virus.* J Virol, 1990. 64(11): p. 5652-5.

386. Tozzini, F., et al., *Simple in vitro methods for titrating feline immunodeficiency virus (FIV) and FIV neutralizing antibodies.* J Virol Methods, 1992. 37(3): p. 241-52.

387. Meers, J., et al., *Feline immunodeficiency virus: quantification in peripheral blood mononuclear cells and isolation from plasma of infected cats.* Arch Virol, 1992. 127(1-4): p. 233-43.

388. Hackett, C.J., *Innate immune activation as a broad-spectrum biodefense strategy: prospects and research challenges.* J Allergy Clin Immunol, 2003. 112(4): p. 686-94.

389. Amlie-Lefond, C., et al., *Innate immunity for biodefense: a strategy whose time has come.* J Allergy Clin Immunol, 2005. 116(6): p. 1334-42.

390. Becker, Y., *The changes in the T helper 1 (Th1) and T helper 2 (Th2) cytokine balance during HIV-1 infection are indicative of an allergic response to viral proteins that may be reversed by Th2 cytokine inhibitors and immune response modifiers--a review and hypothesis.* Virus Genes, 2004. 28(1): p. 5-18.

391. Hofmann-Lehmann, R., et al., *FIV vaccine studies. II. Clinical findings, hematological changes and kinetics of blood lymphocyte subsets.* Vet Immunol Immunopathol, 1995. 46(1-2): p. 115-25.

392. Mazzetti, P., et al., *AIDS vaccination studies using an ex vivo feline immunodeficiency virus model: detailed analysis of the humoral immune response to a protective vaccine.* J Virol, 1999. 73(1): p. 1-10.

393. Nguyen Van, N., et al., *Measurement of cytokine mRNA expression in intestinal biopsies of cats with inflammatory enteropathy using quantitative real-time RT-PCR.* Vet Immunol Immunopathol, 2006. 113(3-4): p. 404-14.

394. Ma, J., et al., *Tumor necrosis factor-alpha responses are depressed and interleukin-6 responses unaltered in feline immunodeficiency virus infected cats.* Vet Immunol Immunopathol, 1995. 46(1-2): p. 35-50.

8. Acknowledgements

I owe a very special debt of gratitude to Prof. Hans Lutz, head of the clinical laboratory of the Vetsuisse faculty in Zürich, for offering me the opportunity to work on this project, as well as for his professional guidance, invaluable support and never-ending optimism throughout my doctoral thesis.

Many thanks are also due to Prof. Mathias Ackermann for his helpful critics and rapid corrections.

I am grateful to Dr. Christiane Juhls and Dr. Manuel Schmidt from Mologen AG, Berlin who supplied us with dSLIM™, for their availability and precious advice in the carrying-out of the various *in vivo* and *in vitro* experiments comprised in this study. I would also like to thank Prof. Oswald Jarret and Dr. Margaret Hosie from the University of Glasgow, Great Britain for their crucial contribution to this project in kindly providing us with the stock of previously-titrated FIV-GL8.

I would further like to express sincere gratitude to all the members of the team working at the clinical laboratory of the Vetsuisse faculty in Zürich for their spontaneous assistance and for the pleasant collegial atmosphere. Particular thanks to Dr. Alice Gomes-Keller and Dr. Ravi Tandon for their patience and expert advice during the cell culture experiments, and to Yousif Ahmed for generous collaboration throughout the project. A special tribute goes to Velia Fornera, our veterinary technician, for her dedication to the well-being of our cats, and for her indispensable help during blood collections.

Acknowledgements

The enthusiastic interest of my office colleagues has been a perpetual source of motivation. A «herzliches Dankeschön» to Claudia and Lea, not only for their precious support, but also for becoming such great friends.

I would also like to extend my sincerest personal thanks to Dr. Christine Poppe, Dr. Kerstin Gabriel and Regula Schwager for their understanding, encouragement and patience during the last phases of my dissertation.

A very special thank you to Anouk, my sister and best friend, whose professional and artistic skills greatly contributed to the remarkable layout of the present manuscript, and whose everlasting energy and dedication have been extremely inspirational.

Finally, I would like to thank my mom and dad for their encouragement in all the projects I have undertaken, and for enabling me to fulfil my dream of becoming a veterinarian. This work would not have been possible without your love and support. Thank you so much!

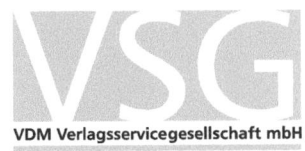

Die VDM Verlagsservicegesellschaft sucht für wissenschaftliche Verlage abgeschlossene und herausragende

Dissertationen, Habilitationen, Diplomarbeiten, Master Theses, Magisterarbeiten usw.

für die kostenlose Publikation als Fachbuch.

Sie verfügen über eine Arbeit, die hohen inhaltlichen und formalen Ansprüchen genügt, und haben Interesse an einer honorarvergüteten Publikation?

Dann senden Sie bitte erste Informationen über sich und Ihre Arbeit per Email an *info@vdm-vsg.de*.

Sie erhalten kurzfristig unser Feedback!

VDM Verlagsservicegesellschaft mbH
Dudweiler Landstr. 99 Telefon +49 681 3720 174
D - 66123 Saarbrücken Fax +49 681 3720 1749

www.vdm-vsg.de

Die VDM Verlagsservicegesellschaft mbH vertritt

 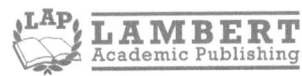 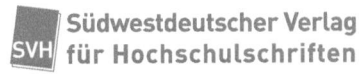

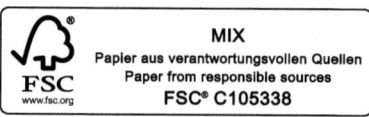

Printed by Books on Demand GmbH, Norderstedt / Germany